LIFE MANAGEMENT SKILLS

MRINAL NAG

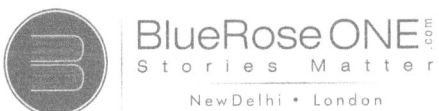

New Delhi • London

BLUEROSE PUBLISHERS
India | U.K.

Copyright © Mrinal Nag 2024

All rights reserved by author. No part of this publication may be reproduced, stored in a retrieval system or transmitted in any form or by any means, electronic, mechanical, photocopying, recording or otherwise, without the prior permission of the author. Although every precaution has been taken to verify the accuracy of the information contained herein, the publisher assumes no responsibility for any errors or omissions. No liability is assumed for damages that may result from the use of information contained within.

BlueRose Publishers takes no responsibility for any damages, losses, or liabilities that may arise from the use or misuse of the information, products, or services provided in this publication.

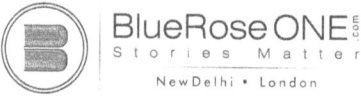

For permissions requests or inquiries regarding this publication, please contact:

BLUEROSE PUBLISHERS
www.BlueRoseONE.com
info@bluerosepublishers.com
+91 8882 898 898
+4407342408967

ISBN: 978-93-5989-427-0

Cover design: Shivam
Typesetting: Namrata Saini

First Edition: August 2024

Dedicated To

The Book, 'LIFE MANAGEMENT SKILLS' is dedicated to those great people, who managed their lives well, became successful, helped the society, were great assets to the society, became famous and lived long.

This book therefore is dedicated to people like Bharat Ratna, Dr A. P. J. Abdul Kalam, a great scientist and former President of India, who was delivering a lecture to the students until his last day at the age of 82; Great Poet and Noble Laureate, Rabindra Nath Tagore, who contributed significantly in the field of Literature till the age of 80; Mr. Peter Drucker, the Father of Modern Management who modernised Business Management and continued teaching at the New York University until the age of 92; and Noble Laureate and Bharat Ratna, Mother Teresa, who diligently served the poor and needy until the age of 87. These remarkable individuals managed their lives well, becoming famous for their enormous contributions to the world and its people.

This book is a humble endeavour to apprise people to learn the nuances of Life Management Skills early in life, so that they all can plan well and learn to manage their lives to have a long, happy, healthy, successful life as well as can help the world and its people for a long time, by taking the inspiration from the great individuals mentioned above.

Foreword

Embarking on the path of Self-Exploration- Guiding life's maze with elegance and intent:

In the vast expanse of human experience, amidst the ebb and flow of life's currents, we find ourselves pondering the essence of our existence. What defines a life of richness and significance? How do we navigate the complexities of our journey with grace and purpose? These are the questions that echo through the corridors of our hearts, transcending the barriers of time and space.

In the captivating pages of 'Life Management Skills', a remarkable book penned by Brigadier. Dr Mrinal Nag, a deep and insightful story emerges, providing valuable direction and enlightenment for those on a journey of self-exploration and development. As I delve into the depths of this remarkable tome, I am struck by its holistic approach towards life, a tapestry woven with threads of introspection, resilience, and boundless optimism.

The journey begins with Chapter I, 'Our Life', where we are invited to contemplate the profound significance of existence itself. Here, amidst reflections on the importance of life and the imperative of planning our journey with intention, we are introduced to the concept of life management- a guiding principle that informs every aspect of our being.

In Chapter II, 'Life is a Marshy Land', we confront the inherent uncertainties and challenges of existence. Through the lens of resilience, we learn to navigate the tumultuous waters of life with courage and determination, emerging stronger and wiser in the face of adversity.

Integral to our journey are the sacred bonds of family and community, as explored in Chapter III, 'Parents and Their Contributions'. Here, we learn to honour the profound role of our elders in shaping our journey, while also contemplating the responsibilities that come with looking after them in their old age.

As we navigate the 'Decider Decade', explored in Chapter IV, we are called upon to seize the opportunities presented to us and chart a course towards a future of fulfilment and purpose. Through astute observations and practical guidance, we learn to harness the transformative power of this pivotal phase in our lives.

Chapter V, 'Skills and Good Practices to Keep the Life on Track', equips us with the tools and practices to stay true to our path amidst life's storms. Here, we glean insights into improving our lives and cultivating the qualities essential for success.

In Chapter VI, 'Some Good Qualities Required to Become Successful', we explore the noble virtues that pave the way towards achievement and fulfilment. Through the cultivation of integrity, perseverance, and compassion, we unlock our full potential and embark on the journey towards success with grace and humility.

The delicate art of managing relationships takes the centre stage in Chapter VII, where we learn to navigate the complexities of human connection with wisdom and compassion. From the bonds of family to the intricacies of love and marriage, we discover the transformative power of authentic connection in fostering harmony and understanding.

In Chapter VIII, 'What is Resilience and How to Convert Failures into Success in Our Lives', we are reminded of the indomitable spirit that resides within each of us, enabling us to rise above life's challenges with unwavering resolve. Through inspiring examples and profound insights, we are empowered to transform setbacks into opportunities for growth and renewal.

The pursuit of holistic development is explored in Chapter IX, where we delve into the essential ingredients for a life of balance and harmony. Here, amidst reflections on the values of education, love, and money, we discover the profound interconnectedness of all aspects of our being.

Chapter X encourages us to contemplate the ultimate aim of our existence- the realisation of our life's goals and aspirations. Through introspection and self-discovery, we uncover the deeper purpose that animates our journey, guiding us towards a future of fulfilment and significance.

As we contemplate the essence of our being in Chapter XI, we are reminded of the sacred contract between self and soul. Here, amidst reflections on the value of time and the importance of time management, we are called upon to honour the gift of life with gratitude and reverence.

In Chapter XII, we confront the realities of stress and mental health, learning to manage the pressures of modern life with resilience and grace. Through the cultivation of mindfulness and self-care, we embark upon a journey towards inner peace and emotional well-being.

As we approach the twilight years of life, Chapter XIII offers insights into planning for retirement with wisdom and foresight. Here, amidst reflections on the preciousness of life and the imperative of cherishing each moment, we are called upon to honour the gift of existence with gratitude and joy.

In the final chapter, we are urged to contemplate the ultimate purpose of our journey- the quest to make our lives a worthy gift for the divine. Through acts of kindness, compassion, and service, we embrace life's fullness with open hearts and minds, offering ourselves as vessels for the expression of divine love and grace.

In conclusion, 'Life Management Skills' serves not only as a profound evidence to the human spirit- an affirmation to our capacity for growth, resilience, and transformation, but also as a sacred roadmap, guiding us towards a life of fulfilment, purpose, and spiritual abundance. Through introspection and the cultivation of sacred relationships, we embark upon a transformative journey, awakening to the profound beauty and significance of each moment, and embracing the fullness of life with open hearts and minds. Through its pages, we are reminded of the timeless truths that guide us on our journey- the importance of self-discovery, the power of resilience, and the imperative of living a life of purpose and significance.

May this extraordinary book serve as a guiding light for all who seek to embrace the fullness of life with courage, resilience, and boundless optimism. As we turn its pages, may we be reminded of the profound beauty and significance of each moment, embracing the journey of life with open hearts and minds.

Dr Sanjay Deshmukh

Formerly, Hon'ble Vice-Chancellor,

University of Mumbai.

About Dr. Sanjay Deshmukh

As a Life Sciences Professor, Dr. Sanjay Deshmukh, the University of Mumbai's youngest-ever full-time Vice-Chancellor, continues to dedicate his service to the institution. He is one of India's widely acknowledged Life Scientists and an important figure in analysing problems arising out of loss of biodiversity, among other front-rank environmental issues. He stands out as the sole University Professor, perhaps in all of India, holding a remarkable accolade as an acknowledged PhD supervisor across five distinct subjects.

Acknowledgements

I would like to acknowledge, thank and express my heartfelt gratitude to my wife Jaya (Dolly) for her genuine love, care, and relentless support in all my endeavours throughout my life, teaching me humility and keeping our fifty years of married life, so enjoyable and happy. She is the epitome of purity, innocence, encouragement and inspiration.

I would also like to thank our sons, Ron and Sundip, for their continuous love and support, which fills a lot of joy and happiness in our lives. Blessed with exceptional qualities and maturity, they are a source of great strength to us.

I would also like to express my thanks and gratitude to our daughters-in-law, Ms. Prachee and Ms. Shaheen, for their love and sincere support, as well as for the happy bonding in the family, which has kept a conducive environment in the family.

Last but not the least, I would like to thank our seven-year-old grand-daughter, Ms. Tiana, for her loving gestures. She is like an angel for us and her presence brings us tremendous amount of joy and happiness.

Source of Inspiration

We have only one life and all of us want it to be a long and happy one. There are some who lived long, became successful, contributed to the welfare of the people of the world. These remarkable individuals not only managed their lives very well but also became a source of inspiration for us all.

Few examples are Mahatma Gandhi, Florence Nightingale, Mother Teresa, Nelson Mandela, Dr A.P.J. Abdul Kalam, Mr. Warren Buffett, who managed their long life very well and became famous for helping the world and its people. Mr. Warren Buffett is an ideal example of our time and is a great Philanthropist who is still serving the people of the world in a noteworthy way.

This book is the result of true inspiration provided by the above-mentioned great figures, who made their lives successful, offered their invaluable services to the humanity, and left their footprints for us all to follow.

Preface

We see many people throughout our lives. People who are happy; unhappy, successful; unsuccessful, enthusiastic, frustrated, energetic, lazy, honest, corrupt etc.

Life is full of uncertainty marked by its highs and lows.

In the absence of any adult or any elder of the family, we cannot plan our lives well, like we cannot take proper advantage during the 'Decider Decade' which refers to the age from 13-14 and 23-24, the most important period in our life, for planning and ensuring a good future. We need the guidance of our parents or a guardian for our proper upbringing so that we sail through the life without much problems, provided we do not indulge in any unwanted habits and can avoid bad company.

If we inculcate few good life management skills, as suggested in this book, we can pave the way for a successful, happy, and healthy life along with making positive contribution to the society as a responsible citizen.

This book on Life Management Skills aims to enlighten and empower the parents to plan the journey of their children's lives well, so that with proper planning, preparation and God's blessings they can lead lives worth living.

In today's technologically advanced era, managing stress has become a very important facet. Many young people, highly paid professionals, are suffering from psychosocial stress. Alarmingly, individuals between the ages of 18 and 40 are dying of heart attacks and some of them are even resorting to suicide because of overwhelming stress.

In a place called Kota, in India, a city known to be a Coaching Factory of India for JEE, NEET and other competitive exams, which are required to qualify for IIT and MBBS course in India, 26 students tragically committed suicide in year 2023 due to the overwhelming stress of passing these important exams. Sadly, the records shows that a lot of students commit suicide every year at Kota for similar reasons.

Learning to manage stress, therefore has become paramount.

At present, there are numerous options available for a child/student. The life of the child is most important, his /her career, though important, is not more important than his /her own life. We love our children more than anything else in this world and we want them to be happy. We must continuously interact with our children and help them bring their stress level down with our love, care and support.

Our children must have enough confidence in us so that they can confide in us for any of their difficulties. The children must know that their success or failure is of much lesser importance than their lives and that at no cost would we want to lose our children just because of their failure in exams/career or any unsuccessful relationship etc.

Our children must know that they are our precious possession and we love them more than anything in this world. They should not sacrifice their lives for any career or anything else.

CHILDREN ARE ALWAYS WELCOME HOME.

This book also provides valuable suggestions regarding essential skills to effectively plan and manage our 'only life' well.

Learning these Life Management Skills would, therefore, help us not only in planning the life of our children and our own but also guide us towards a life that is happy, healthy and fulfilling.

Contents

Introduction 1

Chapter I: Our Life 4
Why life is important to all of us? 4
How to plan our lives? 5
What is Management of life? 8
How to save our life from wrong company, wrong
habits and wrong practices, especially at a young age. 13
Why should we learn to manage our life? 15
Important ingredients of life 17

Chapter II: Life is a Marshy Land, Includes Uncertainties with Ups and Downs 20
How an unfortunate epidemic like Covid-19 affected
our life all over the world 21
Effects of uncertain situations on our Life 24

Chapter III: The Parents and Their Contributions 27
Role of parents in our life 28
Looking After Parents at old age 29

Chapter IV: The Decider Decade 33
Most important Decade of our life 33
Characteristics of this Decade 34
Important Decade for not only Academic Career but
also for other Careers 36
    Sports 36
    Music and Dancing 37
    Character Building 38

Hobbies 40
How to plan to take fullest advantage of this decider decade. 41
Super 6 Years 42
Importance of super 6 years 43
Monitoring children for a few important aspects during super 6 years: 44
    Bad Company 44
    Relationships 45
    Bad Food Habits 45
A Humble Request for The Parents 47

Chapter V: Skills and Good Practices Required to Keep Life on Track 48

We have only one life. 48
Dream big to shape your life. 48
CASE STUDY--1 : Seeing a Big Dream 49
Educate your Mind and Heart, both. 52
Some important skills for a Hassle -Free Life 53
There are 4 types of Attitude :- 56
Learn to Manage Your Emotion 58
Emotional Quotient (EQ) 59
Control your Mind 59
Positive Mind 60
Innovative Mind 61
Creative Mind 61
Some Suggestions to Improve our life 62
    Learn to Adjust 62
    Failure or Rejections is a part of our life. 63
    It is a wonderful life but bad habits can spoil it, choice is yours 64
    Try to become a Skilful Specialist 66

A Moment's Happiness Gained from a
Wrong/Avoidable Source Can Ruin Our Life 67
Select a Career with the Help of Your Parents and
Teachers and Work Towards It.. 68
Be open to Re-Skilling and New Opportunities 69
Accept Change, It is Inevitable.. 69

Chapter VI: Some Good Qualities Required to become Successful.. 71

Communication Skills 71
In social life your good behaviour maintains your
respect and dignity 83

Chapter VII: How to Manage Relationships?.................. 85

a) Relationship with parents. 86
b) Relationship with the Spouse/ Partner........................... 86
c) Relationship with Friends... 87
c) Relationship with the Organizations 88
Romantic Relationship & Vanishing Treasure of Love..... 88
    What is Romance? 89
    Vanishing Treasure of love. 90
    What is Love 91
    Love Letters.. 92
Modern Relationships:... 93
Pandemic offered opportunity for love and prolonged
honeymoon at home. 94
Extra time for Romance During Work From Home
(WFH) 94
Effect of the pandemic in the domestic front affecting
relationship 96
Advantage of being together and increasing love,
due to the Pandemic 97
Work From Home (WFH) and its effect on
Relationship 100

Important Aspects of Work From Home Concept 101
    Employer's perspective 102
    Employee's perspective 102
    Organization's Perspective 104
Renewed family bonding, the biggest contribution of the pandemic 104
We should use our Brain as well as Mind for taking decisions Regarding Relationships and Career without being Emotional. 108
Important Tips for Better Relationships 109

Chapter VIII: What is Resilience and How to Convert Failures into Success in our Life? 113

Few Inspiring Examples: 113
Resilience taught many people to start New Business and Source of Income during The Pandemic 115
Expertise in Data Science and Data Technology 118
Teaching Music and Musical Instruments 118
Human Resousrse Management (HRM) Consultancy Service 119
The power of Resilience developed New Generation of Entrepreneurs with new Start-Ups 122
Resilience Taught us to learn new skills, during Pandemic, for keeping us happy, indoors. 134

Chapter IX: Important Ingredients for Holistic Development. 137

Holistic Development of child is extremely important to be successful in life and to be capable of playing multiple roles in his Personal life as well as Professional Career. 137
Follow Rules, Regulations and laws in our personal and professional life 144
No room for Mediocrity 146

Respect Others Culture, Language and Religion. 146
Be a good citizen of your Country and the World 147
Be a balanced, matured and unbiased person 147
Be empathetic 148
Elevate your next generation to a higher level,
Case Study No-2, Elevate your next generation 148

Chapter X: What is our Life's Goal/Aim? 153
Dharma is righteousness. To be honest and do right
things. 153
What is the Aim of life? 156

Chapter XI: What your life wants from you ? 159
Follow Ethics 159
Work hard to be Successful 159
Try to perform well always, in a 'No mistake'
syndrome 160
If you help people, God will help you 160
Be Properly Qualified, Skilled and be Competent. 161
Look after yourself with Healthy Practices 161

Chapter XII: How to remain Young for a Longer Period? 162
Few Suggested Steps to Remain Young for a Long
Time 164
How to get rid of Smoking and Excessive drinking
to Lead a Healthy Life 168

Chapter XIII: How to manage our Failure and Success in life 176
How to manage our failure 176
How to manage our success 179

Chapter XIV: We have only one Life and it must be a Happy Life. 182

What is Happiness 182
Simple tips to make our life happy 183
How to build a strong personality. 184
    Mental Strength 186
    Physical strength 187
    Emotional Strength 188
Be Smart not to lose any opportunity coming your way. 189
Relation between Materialism and Happiness 189
Role of spirituality in our life 191
Need of Spiritual Quotient, at Senior Level 193
Effect of Spiritual Poverty at Senior Level 194
The additional Mile that you will have to travel to remain ahead of others 194

Chapter XV: A Suggested Road Map for Good Life 197

Some Important Steps To Be Followed To Achieve A Good Life 197
Be Unique, be Different, Nothing is free in this world (Said The Famous, Mr. Jack Ma, Chairman of Alibaba). 198
Learn Soft Skills To Survive 199
Skills and good practices to keep the life on track 206
Role of love, lust, laughter and leisure in our life 208

Chapter XVI: Value of Time and Time Management .. 214

The importance of Time in our life. 214
Ingredients of Time Management 216
Punctuality 216
Multi-Tasking and Punctuality 216
Timely Investments 217
Importance of Finishing Projects on Time 218

Timely Completion of Personal Work and Work of
Our Family..218

Chapter XVII: Value of Education. Love and Money in our life 220

Value of Education in Our Life...220
Value of love in our life..221
Value of Money in our life...222

Chapter XVIII: What is Stress and How to Manage Stress and Mental Health in our life............................... 228

What is Stress and How to Manage Stress........................228
Stress, at times, may be our own creation. 231
How to de-stress yourself..233
What is Mental Health and How to Manage Mental
Health 235
Few Causes of Bad Mental Health and Mental
Depression 236
Some Suggested Remedies...237

Chapter XIX: Express your Gratitude 239

Express your Thanks and Gratitude to God 239
Thank your parents and be grateful to them for your
wonderful upbringing and their sacrifice..........................241
Express your Gratitude to your spouse/partner..............243
Express your gratitude to your Teachers, Mentors
and Seniors...245
We should express our Gratitude to our Children 246

Chapter XX: Planning for a Retired Life 248

How to Plan a Post Retirement Period...............................248
Retired Life Offers Excellent Opportunities to
Enhance our Hobbies 249
More time for physical exercise 251

Few Suggested Steps to enable the Senior Citizens to have a better, busier and more enjoyable life.................... 253

Help the young generation by getting attached to some Educational Institution. 256

Give back to the society 257

Chapter XXI: You Have Only One Life, Respect It, Preserve It, Love It & Live It Appropriately 259

Respect your life 259

Preserve the life 260

Love your life 261

Live appropriately. 263

Chapter XXII: How to Make our Life a Worthy Gift to God 266

Important Aspects Which Can Make Life Worth Living 266

Few Important Steps to Make our Life a Worthy Gift to God 270

Conclusion 271

Introduction

*"What you are is God's gift to you; what you make of yourself is your gift to God." **-George W. Carver***

Our life is the most uncertain aspect that we deal with. Length no one knows, goals evolving to newer goals. But the journey is most uncertain for us. Opportunities are not given, hard work may or may not give results and ultimately, destiny decides the course of our lives.

It is like an enormous sand model, where roads vanish without warning. What appears to be plain ground may lead to towering mountains all of a sudden. Much of it resembles a marshy land except for a few dry spots which ultimately help us to reach our destination and only the lucky ones reach. For many, the road vanishes even before reaching destinations as life may come to an end abruptly.

When a soldier goes to the war, he and his family, his parents, wife and children may have many dreams, the soldier himself may have many dreams, unfinished work, many future plans and worst, most of them believe that he will return. Anybody else may die but he would come back for his family, for his unfinished dreams, to live his full life. But alas, reality can be starkly different. The soldier may not return home from the battle field, or he may return with serious injuries, robbed of his sights, limbs or mobility.

It may happen to any person who may lose life due to an accident. The life is thus uncertain and may be cut short without any pre-warning.

Yet all of us feel and wish that we would, by the grace of God, live a full and meaningful life, i.e., enjoy the whole life and die at an old age touching almost 100, keeping in view the increasing life span across the world.

We should be optimistic and believe that most of us, given that no major war or big accidents occur, would lead a full and meaningful life.

However, life is but a marshy land, full of pot holes, marshy areas, road blocks, obstacles and miseries.

Those of us, who lost our parents at a very young age, know how difficult it is to even survive in this practical and materialistic world. And this happens in many people's lives. Losing a father or a mother or even both at a very young age adds to list of difficulties like financial problems, safety and security problems, grooming and upbringing problem which hinders the natural growth of a child.

With our garnered experience, we have gained an in-depth insight about the characteristics of life and the time-tested routes to success. Though life is full of uncertainty, we can still plan to have a good life for us and for our children.

We can, with our experience, plan our children's life for their better future, guiding them properly through the marshy land of life to a better goal, to higher achievements and to have a happy, healthy, comfortable and peaceful life.

We should try to ensure that our children do not face the similar problems that we faced, and that they become more successful than us leading a safe, secure and more comfortable life. Because we, with our experience, have already learnt the skills necessary to manage our lives and hence, it is our duty to not only improve our lives but also plan and guide our children towards a better and happier life.

It is therefore a huge task to understand the requirements of life and learning the skills essential to manage it, in order to reach our destination. This can only be achieved by travelling and navigating through various marshy areas and road blocks during the hazardous journey of our life . Learning, Life Management Skills, therefore, is extremely important to manage our lives for a more successful and comfortable life and to equip our children with the tools they need for a better, safer, happier, peaceful and comfortable life.

Learning Life Management Skills can be the 'game changer', as we would be able to plan and manage our as well as our children's lives well, to achieve success and happiness.

CHAPTER I

Our Life

Why life is important to all of us?

It is our life. As we grow up, we slowly start learning about life. We see people around us. We see happy and unhappy people; we see successful and failures, we see well-established and struggling people.

We see people with bad habits like excessive drinking, consuming drugs, excessive smoking, spending money in gambling and spoiling their lives and that of their families.

We see noble people helping society, and we also see people engaged in cheating, raping, stealing, and committing all sorts of crimes in society.

Fortunately, we are guided by our parents, teachers, and well-wishers to avoid doing the wrong things or taking inappropriate steps. We are taught to follow the right examples and the right people so that we shape our lives well, enjoy the fruits of good work for a long time, and bring happiness to our parents and family who have contributed most to our lives.

As we start growing, we realise that it is our life and we will have to live it, and we want to live it well.

We start realizing that we have only one life, and we must strive hard to achieve success in our lives to lead a long and happy life.

Our life is our most important possession. We, unfortunately, do not know its length; we cannot predict the disturbances and problems of our lives, yet we try to learn things, try to do things in the right ways, to have a peaceful and happy life.

Not all of us are born into rich families. The majority belong to the middle class, poor class, or even overly poor class. The lives of children born into poor families are extremely difficult. Yet, inspired by happy and successful people around them, they try hard to acquire good education and good habits to become happy and successful in life, lead a happy life, and make their families happy.

It is important how we live our lives and manage to survive through ups and downs to tell ourselves at the end of the day that we had a good life.

Our life ensures our existence; hence it is most important.

How to plan our lives?

It is the parent's prerogative to plan our lives when we are young. They plan initially how to raise a child, his/her upbringing, education, the apparels, food, language, mannerism, etiquette, behaviour inside the house, outside the house etc.

Since education helps in proper upbringing, parents plan the education in school, undergraduate level, and postgraduate level to establish the child's academic career.

If we are fortunate to have our parents supporting us, our standard and quality of education would be good, which would help us throughout our lives.

Unfortunately, many may not receive a good quality education or even basic education. A lot of girls, even in this advanced and civilized world, are not allowed to receive proper, recognized education. And the entire society suffers directly or indirectly from this unfortunate phenomenon. Only an educated mother can teach her child well, the mother being the best teacher for all of us. The more educated the mother, the more the child benefits.

It is therefore very important to provide education to all children, including girls.

In this era of globalization, we are all supposed to be educated, liberal, and broad-minded global citizens. We live in an open society. An educated mother can help a child become mature, balanced, broad-minded, and a good global citizen.

Levels of Education

Planning education for higher classes in school, i.e., IXth, Xth, XIth, XIIth level (including AS and A Levels), is extremely important for higher studies and choosing the proper professional line.

Teachers, particularly education counsellors, can help the parents and the child a lot at this stage.

The professional line and requirements of higher education, therefore, must be planned well in advance, keeping in view the child's area of interest. It is of no use if a child is pushed into experiments. There are quite a few examples where students have left the studies of engineering, medicine, etc., even in the 3rd or 4th year because they felt they were not interested in the curriculum.

The higher education required for a particular profession needs a particular mindset, self-interest, and passion. It must be part of the child's dream to be what his parents, teachers, or even peers want him or her to be, or else the entire effort would become a costly and avoidable disaster.

In India, we have various boards of education, like State Boards, CBSE, ICSE, IB, etc, and each curriculum is different, and the standard of education is also different. There is a visible difference between students of State Boards (Vernacular Medium) and International Baccalaureate (IB), (English Medium).

The bright and talented students from the State Boards, at times, do not get the opportunities that the students from IB get, due to reasons known to all of us.

Another important aspect of planning the life of a child is his or her birthplace. Students from rural areas do not have the facilities, especially in developing countries, that students from urban areas do. As a result, students from rural areas are less equipped to face the modern and digital world.

The poor financial conditions, lack of communication skills, rural lifestyle, and lack of modern facilities also put the students of rural areas at a disadvantage compared to the students of urban areas. Career planning for rural students is often difficult due to a lack of facilities in rural areas.

For example, India is a vast country with 1.4 billion people. 65% of whom reside in rural areas. The number of students deprived of good opportunities and facilities is large. This is a problem for many other countries with a vast rural population, where many bright and talented students with good potential lack the facilities to develop properly.

It is therefore very important that all facilities, such as Wi-Fi, the Internet, digital technology, and qualified teachers, be made available in every part of the country. It is also important that a Common National Curriculum , incorporating an Updated International Curriculum, be taught in the entire country at the secondary, higher secondary, undergraduate, and postgraduate levels, to provide similar education to all students, at all levels, so that all students study similar curriculum, irrespective of the place they belong to and have similar advantage , which students of Urban Areas enjoy.

A modern, updated, Industry-Related, Research-Oriented syllabus, including new and relevant subjects, practical projects, skill-based workshops, internships, should be adopted, which will make the students Industry/Market ready and employable. Syllabus should be updated every three years, to remain relevant.

Good Quality of Education is very important for the Nation Building.

What is Management of life?

Our life has four stages:

1. Childhood & Adolescence

2. Young Adult Age

3. Middle Age

4. Old Age

Childhood & Adolescence Stage:

Our childhood stage, and until we arrive at adulthood via period of adolescence, is managed and nurtured by our parents. Their love, care, guidance, and planning ensure our safety, security, and proper upbringing.

Our parents sacrifice a lot during this growing-up period to keep us happy, healthy, safe, and secure. They take entire responsibility for food, shelter, education, and medical emergencies. They teach us values that stay with us throughout our lives.

In fact, our parents, at this stage, try to plan our proper development, higher education, and academic as well as professional career.

Even the poorest parents aim to bring up their children with high dreams. For example, a mother, the wife of a rickshaw puller, dreams of making her son a doctor or an engineer when he grows up. They may not be able to afford good school or college, but they hold onto their dream as a secret desire in their hearts, wishing for a miracle to happen so that they can afford good education and upbringing for their child.

Proper guidance during adolescence is extremely important. A lot of school and college dropouts happen at this stage. Many children get into wrong habits of smoking, or drinking, etc. Additionally, a lot of students, during this stage, get into relationships with opposite sex and become emotionally involved, deviating from their goals to achieve success in life. As children at this stage are very emotional and vulnerable, they struggle to tackle multiple problems from multiple angles leading to a rising number of suicide cases. These growing kids need our help.

Guidance from parents, good friends, and teachers can play a very important role in shaping one's life at this stage, especially in keeping children on the proper track so that they are not influenced by wrong, disgruntled, or frustrated people who have given up on their dreams, future, and life. There are many lazy, mischievous, and unsuccessful people in the society. Without friends, these spoilt lot often try to influence teenagers to get into avoidable and wrong habits. "A man is known by the company he keeps" is an important quote that must be understood by the young people. Wrong company may spoil your life.

The adolescence period is when a child reaches of puberty. A child undergoes many changes in their body, mind, and voice, etc. A girl child has to learn to manage menstruation at this stage, which can cause a lot of mental and physical stress. There are significant hormonal and physical changes that occur in a girl's body during this time. Irregular menstruation can create various peculiar physical changes in a girl's body, including unwanted obesity, leading to both physical and mental stress and discomfort. Parents, particularly the mother, can be a great help to a girl child at this stage.

Change in voice quality will be major change in a boy, apart from growing beard and moustache on the face, a significant transformation as a boy slowly develops into a man. It is very important to note that, as a growing boy, one should remain focused, listen to parents and teachers, who are true friends, and avoid bad company to grow up naturally and properly.

Young Adult Age

This stage of our life is extremely important for all of us. We either make it or break it. From the age of 18 onwards, we are adults. We pursue higher education in professional courses like Medicine, Engineering etc. Academic results at this stage are very important as good results open many doors to good career opportunities for us.

Young adulthood, especially the age from 18 to 40, is extremely important as we strive to finish our professional courses, Masters, PhDs, etc. We try to join good industries/corporate offices to start a strong and progressive professional career.

Any mistake or offence at this stage would lead to a lot of embarrassment as we are adults. Even avoidable language written in an e-mail can cause a of lot of embarrassment for oneself and the family.

A moment's mistake, due to youthful exuberance and lack of maturity, can lead to punishment under the law.

People who are focused, dedicated, and eager may lay a solid foundation for their long-term success during this period.

Young adulthood also brings significant adjustments to our lives. People prefer to settle down, marry, purchase property, automobiles, and generally enjoy their lives.

This is the period when individuals have children, take care of their elderly parents (if they still live together), invest for the future, and strive to provide a pleasant life for their families. This stage of life is also critical for establishing oneself successfully in a professional career. The work-life balance becomes increasingly vital. Some household comforts may need to be sacrificed in order to advance in one's professional life.

This phase requires patience, and maturity to handle basic needs of life.   More so, if both the partners are working then work would keep them away from home for a long time, at times, even neglecting children and elderly parents. Traveling for senior professionals is also a constant source of unpleasantness in the family, when one may miss important events like marriage anniversaries, children's birthday, and parent-teacher meetings in schools etc. Frequent travels and busy schedule in office, at times, can create a lot of disturbance and misunderstanding in family life, especially during this stage of life.

Middle Age

In present era, age 40 to 60 are considered middle age due to increasing longevity and life span

Middle age brings a lot of added responsibilities in everyone's life. Children pursue higher education, which can be a very expensive affair, while parents in advanced age group would be needing more attention especially medical assistance. On the professional front, we reach pinnacle of our career which is very demanding regarding time, own mental and physical energy, and maturity to solve complex professional matters. People may be married for 20/25 years and since the children are grown-up, they may be out of home for higher education or even jobs. The spouse, who is not working may demand more time / more company, as she/ he may feel lonely at home staying alone the entire day, which is seen quite often as our family now mostly consists of husband, wife, and the children only. The middle age is quite demanding from all angles, with increased responsibilities. Furthermore, it also leads to Retirement where the income decreases but the responsibilities such as children's higher education, marriages, EMI of house continue.

Old Age

Known to be the final stage of our life, in the modern era, old age typically starts around 60 or 65 and ends when the God almighty wants it to end. It simply depends on individual's habits, health, and destiny. There are lot of people now who live beyond 90 and even surpass 100 years of age.

Japan has '100 plus years club' where people more than 100 years of age are members.

Old age can be likened to dealing with an old machine, made by God, each machine is different and in most cases people who maintain their body machine well with regular physical exercise, good habits like no smoking, no drinking or less drinking, live a healthy life. With good and positive mindset as well as ethical behaviour, one commits lesser mistakes in life.

He does not harm or cheat others, and lives a longer lifespan with fewer tension and worries.

One thing is clear: a good person with the above-mentioned qualities lives a happy life, and whether he or she lives up to 100 years or not, he or she dies as a happy and content person.

Old age is the stage where a person has fewer responsibilities, with the children often settled and one is free from official duties, allowing more personal time. This is an opportunity where one should contribute to the society in meaningful ways. Giving back to society has no age limit. Old age must be spent in a planned manner, as there are numerous fulfilling activities to perform.

Elderly people possess valuable experience and knowledge, they are assets to the society. They may spend their time teaching underprivileged children, volunteering for NGOs, or offering charitable services. They can also help some poor families financially, as per their own capacity.

One must remain active and engaged even in old age. Basic physical activities will keep us physically fit, as there may not be anyone to look after us if we fall sick. Every country does not have the access to facilities for free medical attention. In most cases, the growing children would be staying abroad due to work or business, and quite often, elderly parents are left alone in their houses, relying on neighbours, housing societies, and luck for support. Being active in old age, offering service to society, maintaining physical fitness, and doing good to people would lead to a satisfying conclusion to our lives.

How to save our life from wrong company, wrong habits and wrong practices, especially at a young age.

Throughout our lives, we meet various types of people in our life, spanning from those disinterested in life, happy, unhappy, successful, unsuccessful, frustrated, disgruntled, balanced, and imbalanced, as well as decent and indecent.

Each person has his own reasons to behave the way he behaves. The company of a failure will gradually draw us into a similar pattern, as one gets used to it. We have to very carefully, swim away from those hurdles. A successful person will encourage and inspire us to strive for success. A frustrated man will be unhappy and cribbing but an achiever will always be happy, energetic, and positive.

To safeguard ourselves, we must be smart to stay clear from the failures, frustrated and unhappy people as well as individuals with bad habits and bad practices such as excessive smoking, heavy drinking, gambling, and people who fail in the same class year after year, as they have no ambition.

Following the values taught by our parents, teachers, remaining engaged in sports and physical activities and hobbies would keep us away from negative influences. Sports and physical activities would keep us fit and energetic and good hobbies like music, playing instruments or reading would keep us suitably engaged in young age. We can thus remain away from the sway of bad company and avoid doing wrong things.

Once a child starts playing outdoor games like football, cricket, basketball, and hockey, he plays for long hours, for which he needs strength and stamina hence, he does not pick up bad habits like smoking, and drinking, etc. He learns good things like team spirit, team building, sportsman's spirit, leadership, patience, tolerance, camaraderie etc., which are good qualities for a person. He thus becomes a matured, balanced and well-behaved person, who dreams to do well in life and does not get influenced by any disgruntled person.

If a child adopts a hobby such as music, whether it's singing or playing musical instruments, then he becomes engrossed in practice, rehearsals, for long hour. This does not give him time to mix with people who are idle or doing unwanted things. Parents should spend more time with their children, and pay attention to them so that they can help their children avoid bad company. Parent's love, affection and quality time spent together, can help a child to develop naturally, avoiding harmful influence.

Why should we learn to manage our life?

The term "Management" refers to the process of getting the work or the task done that is required for achieving the goals of an organization, in an efficient and effective measures.

According to Henri Fayol, the functions of business management include planning, organizing, staffing, directing and controlling.

Management in our life is also very important. It also includes all aspects of the business management. Parents and growing children who grasp this concept often achieve the goals in their life and become successful.

It is an important task of every parent to meticulously plan and organize their child's life and career. The child needs constant guidance, direction, and oversight of parents until they are big and matured enough to take on the responsibility for their own growth.

All of us must understand that it is our duty to work hard, utilizing our intelligence and skills to uplift the next generation.

While all of us are not born into wealth, or enjoy the same privileges and resources, it remains our duty and responsibility to establish ourselves in life and provide all the facilities to the next generation, to change their life style, making them more comfortable so that they can be proud of us.

It is of no use blaming our parents or past generation, if we do not have a comfortable life, because the parents were poor. Even rich parents can become poor overnight, due to various circumstances like earthquake, political disturbance, floods, partition of a country (as happened in India in 1947), etc. Instead, we should be determined to do well in life to make our parents and elders happier and more comfortable by achieving our goals and becoming successful.

Managing our life, is therefore very important.

Every child, between the ages of 15 to 16, must understand several vital life lessons:

- Parents may or may not be available for long. Life is most uncertain and one should be ready for the worse.

- The "Decider Decade" between the age of 13/14 to 23/24, is very important for everybody. We must work hard, study hard to fulfil our dreams, achieve our goal. If we relax now or indulge in enjoyment now, then we will miss the opportunities and we may not be successful in life.

- Typical forms of entertainment like peer's company, picnics, movies, cyber games etc. can all wait. These few years from 13/14 to 23/24 are most important for our career and success in life.

- It is our life and parents may or may not be able to guide us all the time. But every child must understand that since it is his life, he has to work hard to succeed. He has to learn to manage his own life to achieve his dreams and succeed for the comfort as well as well-being of the future generations.

- Learning to manage our life is therefore very important.

Important ingredients of life

Our life is a complex journey with a few important ingredients, one should not lose sight of. These are:

1. Childhood – Growing under parent's care.

2. Adolescences – growing stage of life, knowing and learning new and strange things about life.

3. Change in voice quality, change in the physical appearance, especially in girls, knowing peculiarities of body, normal changes, new experience like menstruation for girls and managing menstruation, development of attraction towards opposite sex etc.

4. Adulthood –A grownup person, finishing stage of studies, joining job or business, getting the taste of economic independence because of own income.

5. Experience of relationships, which may lead to marriage and then may lead to having own children. Taste of own domestic life with own spouse, children etc., understanding responsibilities of the family and the organization in which we work.

Few Important aspects:

a) Experience about relationship, friends, spouse.

b) Trying to learn to maintain the balance between work and family life.

c) Responsibility of bringing up children.

d) Constant hard work and endeavour to excel in career.

e) Trying to learn about how to get used to the more work pressure at senior level and stressful domestic life because of the demands of family life and the professional career.

Important aspects about domestic life and own old age:

1. Domestic needs and urge to buy properties and other costly items and bearing pressure of EMIs / Economic hardships.
2. Bearing the high cost of children's higher education.
3. Looking after old parents
4. Own retirement and trying to manage a retired life and expenses.
5. Own old age, managing own health, medical bills and psychological and physical difficulties.
6. Facing and getting used to reduced importance, increasing physical and medical problems, neglect, at times facing criticism from own people for less success/achievement and helplessness, even loneliness of own old age which one has to bear, suffering silently till the last day.

These ingredients are common to almost all people barring very few exceptions.

There are good days and bad days, happy times, unhappy times, days when you are in high demand, everyone wants to talk to you, meet you, and there will days when people will ignore you, avoid you, even your own people won't be happy to meet you, and may criticize you. That is life and all these spicy ingredients are a part of our beautiful platter called life.

We must prepare ourselves for it, we have to face it, tolerate it, and digest it like a dose of Quinine (a bitter pill).

As the famous Indian Ghazal singer, Mr. Jagjit Singh, expressed in his famous Ghazal "Hamsafar Hota Koi To Baant Lete Duriaan"------ "Haadso ki bhir hai, chalta hua yeh karwan, Zindegi ka naam hai–Laachaarian -Majburian.", which may mean, and I may not be entirely correct in translating this, however the meaning is " The long journey of our life, with lots of people, are full of accidents and bad incidents. The name of life is helplessness and being compelled by the situations destined for us."

We have no choice, even emperors, kings, queens, presidents, and prime ministers, face these similar problems in life just as a common man faces. Money, power and status cannot change the destiny of a person. Life is a tough journey for all of us equally.

But this suffering can be reduced provided we are prepared to spend our life properly and purposefully. The number of accidents and bad incidents can be reduced if we learn to be cautious and manage our lives carefully.

This book is a humble endeavour to teach us Life Management Skills which will equip us to go through the complex journey of life with great comfort and would enable us to face the end, well, with the blessings of God.

CHAPTER II

Life is a Marshy Land, Includes Uncertainties with Ups and Downs

Our life is akin to a Marshy Land. There are dry roads, good paths, and rocky terrains, as well as sinking areas that threaten to spoil our journey.

In our early days, parents take care of us, look after us, and guide us along smooth, dry path. We enjoy our childhood the most because of our parents. We don't have to think; we don't have to worry. The path is full of love, affection, safety, security, and growth. We don't have to worry about food, clothing, shelter, etc. Parents' guide us forward, holding our hands, and we enjoy the best time of life during childhood.

But there are quite a few who lose their parents quite early in life. Losing both parents can make you feel almost like an orphan. While you may have your sisters and brothers, but no one can take the place of your parents. Life, all of a sudden, becomes hell; you have to survive without your parent's help leaving you at the mercy of others. Even your sisters and brothers, especially the ones younger than you, also suffer like you. You have to not only survive, but also, look after the younger ones and as a result, your education and own well-being often take a back seat. If you have an elder brother or sister, you are lucky, particularly an elder brother, who can, in some way, look after the family.

Again, you are indeed fortunate if you have a home and other assets as your elder brother can provide some level of support for the family.

However, we see a lot of tragic cases where parents die of a car accident, plane crash, or epidemic like COVID-19, etc. Such incidents can devastate even the most stable family overnight.

In such circumstances, your dreams, your welfare, and that of your siblings suffer profoundly.

In another scenario, parents may be alive and looking after their child, but the child meets with a serious accident while riding a motorbike and loses both legs drastically altering his life. He has to learn to live with imputed legs. His confidence, dreams, and even dignity become a big challenge.

As we grow up, completing our studies, we try to settle down with a good job, we may get married and have children. We enjoy a nice little family with our spouse and kids. If our spouse also works in any organization, we have better financial conditions, more disposable income, more materialistic happiness like a better car, a bigger house, a better children's education, etc. Everything may go well, but all of a sudden, there may be an economic meltdown in the world, like it happened in 2007–2009 (due to the subprime problem) or in 2020–21, a situation like COVID-19, when the world came to standstill. Business activities stopped, companies shut shops, people lost their jobs, and in the worst case, both husband and wife lost their jobs.

How an unfortunate epidemic like Covid-19 affected our life all over the world

Covid-19 was like a vast marshy area in our lives, where everyone suffered for 2 years. Many people lost their lives, and countless families suffered. The pandemic suddenly impacted everyone's life throughout the world. People were getting infected and becoming almost untouchable. Doctors also suffered immensely while treating the sick patients. Relatives were kept away, they were not allowed to go near dead bodies, unable to bid farewell and thousands were dying every day. No proper medicines or vaccine were available. Millions of patients even in advanced countries like US succumbed to the virus.

Normal patients suffering from hypertension, diabetes, heart ailments, pneumonia, viral fever etc. could not visit any hospital. Even the operations/surgeries were postponed as the hospitals were full of Covid patients. Cancer patient needing urgent treatment could not go to hospital. Even accident cases, needing immediate surgery, had a tough time to get treatment. The entire world had stopped suddenly. Normal life was totally disturbed in an unpredicted situation like Covid-19 overnight. The industries were shut, business stopped, offices were closed, and many bread earners of the families lost their jobs.

People were confined to their homes. People were scared of the daily death toll. Our so called life, even for well settled people got disturbed beyond imagination. Kings, Queens, CEOs, MDs, Celebrities also died, hence common people were very scared.

Covid-19, stopped the functioning of the world and people at the bottom of the pyramid, the daily wage earners, and poor people, suffered most, as all business activities had stopped.

Some industries which were badly affected were as follows:

- Airlines
- Shipping and luxury liners
- Hospitality including hotel and restaurants

- Transportation including Trains, road transport, taxies, buses, tourist buses etc.
- Shopping malls, shops etc.
- Entertainment industries including film Industries, multiplexes, theatres, cinema halls.
- Food industries, including small eateries
- Travel industry, travel agencies etc.
- Education sector all schools, and colleges and universities were shut
- Lot of small and cottage industries closed down due to no/less demand
- Real estates and infrastructure industries
- Railways, Metros
- All offices were closed. Work From Home (WFH), started in most of the organizations.
- Print media suffered badly as people stopped taking newspapers, magazines etc.
- Agriculture/Farming were affected as a lot of labourers went back to their native place.

As a result of the industries getting closed, countless people throughout the world lost jobs all of a sudden, which increased their misery as they were unable to pay their monthly EMIs and fees for school-going or college-going children. Maintaining the family alone had become a difficult task.

Children could not play outside, earning members got stuck at home. Every house almost became like a jail as the occupants got confined within the house 24/7. It was as if all of us got entangled in the shifting sands of a marshy land.

The entire world was stunned, shocked, worried, scared, and helpless because of an extremely contagious and dangerous disease known as COVID-19, which originated in China.

The people of both rich countries and poor countries suffered alike, as governments struggled to improve the medical infrastructure and increase the numbers of medical staff to tackle the unpredicted health fiasco. This experience was unique, unimaginable, and extremely scary for all of us.

So, a normal life can also be disturbed due to an unforeseen event, like COVID-19.

In the 20th century, around 1918 or 1919, the Spanish flu also created a similar situation for many. But COVID-19 was even worse.

Our lives are therefore somewhat like a Marshy Land; we may encounter shifting sands at times, and only our power of resilience can get us back to a stable position.

Effects of uncertain situations on our Life

1. Covid-19, had a very bad effect on all of us. All of us suffered from bad economic conditions. The burden of EMIs on Car/House etc, became overwhelming. This kind of situation has happened in the past and may even be repeated in the future. This part of life resembles traversing through a marshy area, and it takes time and a lot of effort to overcome this situation and survive.

2. Another challenging situation a person may face in his life, is when his wife is pregnant and his old parents need medical attention, treatment, medicine, and even surgery, the monthly expenditure is too much to handle, and the only bread earner loses his job due to the downsizing of the company. He may also face problems like relocation from his job, his own bad health condition, etc., which may add more misery to his life.

3. A similar situation can also happen to a businessman when, all of a sudden, business earnings drop because of new competitors in similar business with better quality and efficiency, and new technology. The result is the same, financial hardship for himself and his family. There are a lot of businessmen who suffer like this and try to start some other business to re-establish themselves. But the family goes through a very bad time and struggles.

During Covid-19, many businesses suffered severe setbacks. Airlines, travel and tourism, hotels and restaurants, malls and theatres, small shops, transportation, etc., and a lot of industries and business houses had to shut down. Many businessmen went bankrupt, and their families suffered very badly. Overnight, some rich people became poor.

This experience mirrors travelling through marshy terrains in our life, which is full of uncertain, unknown, and unplanned activities.

Our lives can thus be compared to a marshy land, and we must be very careful about choosing our path, be ready for alternative routes, be flexible, be resilient, be ready to face unforeseen eventualities, and despite that, be able to complete this uncertain, complex, yet enjoyable journey of our lives.

Those of us who are fortunate enough to lead a normal life by the grace of God, must thank the divine every day.

We should try to learn certain skills as mentioned below:

- To stay alive by avoiding risks of rash driving and other avoidable risks.
- To educate and update ourselves to become relevant and properly qualified

- To learn skills required in the present era of industries like AI, 3D/4D Printing, Robotics, Block Chain, new code languages like Python, JavaScript, Typescript etc.
- To learn social skills in order to survive in the society
- Learn to avoid bad influence of some known people who might drag us to bad habits or wrong path, leading to a journey akin to a marshy land.
- To survive in situations like Covid-19

CHAPTER III

The Parents and Their Contributions

Our life starts when we are born from our mother's womb. When we begin as helpless human beings, who cannot speak, stand or are unable to do anything for ourselves.

But a human life has started, and the parents, especially the mother, looks after the child with utmost attention, tremendous love, and care. She spends every second with the child looking after the child, feeding the child with her own breast milk and changing nappies even at the middle of the night when everyone else in the house is sleeping.

The parents, especially the mother, is therefore very important in our lives, as a helpless, unaware child would never know what the mother has done for him/her and what sacrifices she has made, ignoring her own comfort, sleep and well-being. A mother experiences a rebirth when her baby is born. Many mothers died in past while delivering a baby, including Queen Mumtaz, the queen of Mughal Emperor Shah Jahan, who died just after delivery of the 14th child, due to weakness and bad health. Emperor Shah Jahan constructed the famous Taj Mahal at Agra, in India, in her memory. An ideal example of expression of love, people from all over the world visit this 'Symbol of Love' every year.

We all, whether a common man, millionaire, billionaire, king, emperor, queen, prime minister, or president, are born helpless. The baby needs help and who helps? The mother and father, i.e., the parents, help. In case of a single parent, she/he helps until the child becomes a grown-up and independent person. Even when a child grows up, parents still remain concerned about the child, as they love him/her so much. When child is sick, the mother and father do not sleep the whole night, as they look after the child. Parents become unhappy if a grown-up child is unhappy for any reason. Parents support the child during his/her struggling period because parents are the best friends of a child. Parents are our permanent friends. Parents love their children more than they love themselves.

Role of parents in our life

Parents, particularly the mother, does a lot to ensure that the infant is adequately cared for, protected, nourished, and secured from all sides. She never takes her eyes off the baby. As the child grows, both the mother and father take great care in raising the child. They are particularly concerned with the child's well-being, education, health, cleanliness, sanitation, and nutrition.

Parents want to see their child grow up and succeed in life, even better than themselves. As a result, parents work hard to feed the child properly, send him/her to a decent school, and satisfy all of the child's needs just to see a grin on his/her face.

We all must know that our parents have sacrificed a lot, working very hard for our proper growth, sacrificed their own comfort, leisure and happiness. We must realize that parents are the best friends in the world and not fair-weather friends like many we think are our best friends.

We, therefore, should not forget to do our part when our parents become old. As children, we needed them while growing up, but they may need us when they are old and may need help.

Parent's contribution in our life is enormous; without their help, we would not be in a position that we enjoy today.

We need our parent's help when we are very young, and likewise, parents may need our help when they are old. We must remember to help them when they need it. Our careers, important assignments, engagements, and family commitments are important, but we must understand that parents have no one without us. We must ensure to help them and be with them, even at the cost of criticism from the professional or domestic front because they are our parents. No one knows more about their contribution in our lives than us.

Our duty bound and positive approach also will teach our children to choose the correct priorities in life.

Our duties towards our parents will teach our children the importance of family bonding. Children learn about values from us, and thus the legacy continues.

A happy family is a huge support and a great source of happiness, and parents are the anchor of a family.

Looking After Parents at old age

Parents look after us from the day we are born. In fact, they, especially the mother, looks after us even when we are in the womb. She sacrifices many things, enduring bad health, morning sickness, uneasiness, extra weight, difficulty in movement, limitation of food intake, and the danger of childbirth.

By the time we are well settled and in our 40s to 50s, our parents are old.

We may be staying in another city for work, with both husband and wife working and staying very busy. Meanwhile, the old parents may be staying in the old house, in the original place, all by themselves. Parents in their 70s & 80s are very old and face numerous problems including health issues, housework, cooking, shopping, safety, security, and boredom. They wait for the children, now grown up, to come & stay with them. They want to spend time with their grandchildren.

But in reality, this does not happen nowadays. The joint family system has disappeared. Old parents stay by themselves and somehow pass their time. They go to the hospital themselves, do the household work, and manage to spend a boring life. The grown-up children have their own families and children and remain busy with their professional and domestic work. The grown-up children, at times, may be too busy to meet the parents often and if they live aboard, they visit after long intervals.

Parent's love, affection, and all the sacrifices they make for children remain embedded in their hearts and become a big source of pain if neglected by their children. Fortunately, the number of such children is very less.

Parents, in their old age, depend on their grown-up children.

All of us must, therefore, realize that it is our responsibility to look after the parents who did so much and sacrificed so much to make us well-established and happy. Parents also keep their assets, properties and possessions for us to enjoy life more. We must ensure that our beloved parents are confident of our help, just as we were always confident of their help whenever we needed it. We should assure them of our support at all times because we also love them dearly. Parents are like God to all of us, who love us so much. Parent's blessings are great assets in our life, and to understand this, one only needs to ask someone who grew up without parent's love and care.

Disrespecting or neglecting parents is akin to disrespecting or neglecting God.

The worst experience for our parents is when one of them passes away, leaving the other alone, sometimes for several more years. Quite often, the old mom/dad is kept in an old age home.

In my opinion, this is an incorrect decision by the children. After all their love and sacrifice, parents do not deserve to stay in an old age home. Children should be mature and responsible enough to look after their parents when they are helpless.

Any advice from friends, relatives, or even a spouse to keep a single parent in an old age home must be ignored by the children. After all, they are your parents, and you, as their children must look after them. And if someone is unhappy with your decision, tell them to think about their own parents, as they also deserve good treatment.

Fortunately, there are plenty of examples where young generations have displayed genuine love for parents and grandparents. The present generation, in my opinion, is very responsible, caring and loving. They care for their parents a lot.

I know one of my girl students who stayed back in India just to be with her grandmother while her parents were in the US. She was studying MBA and looked after her grandmother with a helping hand at the hose.

I also know of a girl who flew down from London to Mumbai to meet and look after her seriously ill grandmother.

The example set by our two sons, Ron and Sundip, is also worth mentioning. They looked after me extremely well when I recently had a head surgery. Both sons, along with their wives, were a great help to me and my wife, who was under a lot of stress. My wife and I are very fortunate to have such good children. I wish all children were as responsible, loving and caring.

These examples are very inspiring and make senior citizens and especially all parents happy.

All children and grandchildren love their parents and grandparents. Some of them change, unfortunately, after their marriage and when they have their own family. Especially, children who are settled abroad and have their own family are, at times, unable to look after their parents due to distance, busy office schedules, and family commitments. They convey their love by greeting on 'Mother's Day' or 'Father's Day', whereas the parents wait anxiously to meet them.

We must all understand that today's young ones will become old parents with similar problems after some time. Treating our old parents well now will encourage and inspire our own children to treat us the same way when the time comes.

CHAPTER IV

The Decider Decade

Most important Decade of our life

It is extremely important for all of us, especially the young ones, to understand that the decade from 13/14 years to 23/24 years is the most important period of our life.

Children or students at the age of 13/14 are at the threshold of stepping into higher education. They face important exams in the next few years and the result of these exams determines their academic career, which in turn leads to their professional career in the future. They typically finish their Graduation by 20/21 and Master's degree by 23/24 if they continue their studies after Graduation. If interested in pursuing a Ph.D., they can finish by 26/27 years, especially with the help of internet facilities.

Children and students who are focused, determined, resilient, and work hard to fulfil their dreams, become successful and enjoy their lives in the future. However, those who do not understand the value of the decade of 13/14 to 23/24 years, of their lives, suffer throughout their lives.

There is a famous saying in the army: "Soldiers who sweat more during peace time (i.e., train hard during peace time) bleed less during the war." This is true in our lives as well. The students and children who work hard during this decade to achieve their goals suffer less in real life.

Human beings have a limited lifespan. Though everyone hopes to live for 100 years, and we often receive blessings or bless young ones to live for 100 years, in reality, the lifespan of a person remains uncertain. On average, a person lives for 70–80 years, approximately.

In this short span of life, a person experiences childhood, adulthood, middle age, and old age.

Out of 70 or 80 years, one decade is extremely important because it determines the course of our lives. It is the decade that, if planned and worked properly, makes a person successful in life. This critical decade spans from 13/14 years to 23/24 years.

It is my humble endeavour to apprise everyone, especially the young ones and their parents, about the importance of this decade in our lives so that we do not miss the bus.

The decade of 10 years, from 13/14 to 23/24 years, is the most important period of our lives. Proper planning and methodical as well as timely implementation can make this decade from 13/14 years to 23/24 years most fruitful, which will eventually determine the course of our lives. But alas, people who do not understand the importance of this decade will struggle throughout their lives due to a lack of vision and timely effort.

Characteristics of this Decade

Children at the age of 13/14 years are growing and are mostly at the threshold of stepping into higher education. At this stage, they are typically at the level of secondary education. As teenagers with less experience of life and maturity, they are still under the guidance of their parents.

The important characteristics of the decade are as follows:

At the age of 13, a child is in grade 7th or 8th. As he completes 13th year and steps in 14th year, he is in grade 8th or 9th, as prevalent in India at present. The planning for higher education starts at this stage. A child begins to take specific subjects from grade 9th, depending on his choice of further studies. If the child wants to pursue studies in engineering or medicine, he chooses science subjects like Physics, Chemistry, Maths and Biology. If the child prefers the commerce stream or arts (literature) stream, he chooses non-science subjects like Economics, Accounts, History, Geography, Sociology, Philosophy, and languages like Hindi/ English Literature.

Parents, at this stage, play a crucial role in deciding about a child's future course of education, like for example, in India, there are various educational boards like State Boards, CBSE, ICSE and IB etc, parents enrol their children in schools under any of these boards, keeping in view the academic career aspirations of the child.

As we know CBSE & ICSE Boards, in India, are good for Engineering and Medicine Education in India. Whereas, if a child wants to pursue his studies abroad with the ultimate aim of doing post-graduation or Ph.D. in any reputed Foreign University, then IB curriculum would be very beneficial. This decision should be taken when the child is 13/14 years old.

The moment such decisions are taken, especially in countries like India and Indian sub-continent, parents often enrol their children in various coaching classes or institutes for preparation to qualify for the entrance exams. For example, in India, to get admission in IIT, the premier institute for engineering, they have to clear JEE which is a tough exam. Qualifying in this exam allows a student to get admission in any of the IITs. The similar entrance exam like NEET is there for medical courses like MBBS.

These entrance exams are taken after 12th Grade. A child is about 17 / 18 at this stage. He has to study hard for the next 4 / 5 years to qualify to be an Engineer or a Doctor. Likewise, there is an entrance exam for 5-year LLB course.

Students who follow the regular course of education typically go for a 4-year degree course, to qualify as BA, BSc, or B.COM graduates. A few students interested in further studies go on to obtain master's degree. Children in normal course, complete graduation by 20/21 years. Those who opt for further higher studies pursue their master's in Arts, Science, or Management subjects for the next 2 years and finish post-graduation by about 23/24 years. It is, therefore, seen that a proper planning has to be done for a child's academic career from the age of 13/14 and continue through to 23/24 years. The decade, 13/14 to 23/24 years, therefore is very crucial, and vital for child's academic career which in turn helps in building his professional career in the future.

Very few choose to do a Ph.D. immediately after completing their master's degree, and that may take 3 to 5 years more. However, the time taken to complete Ph. D, has reduced now due to the advancements in the internet and the information technology.

Important Decade for not only Academic Career but also for other Careers

The Decider Decade is important for all careers, in addition to Academic Career, since talented children start their career in many other fields from the age of 13/14.

Sports

This decade is also crucial for a sportsperson. Like academics, the talented sports personnel must note and understand their potential and passion and build on it. Great cricketers like

Bharat Ratna Sachin Tendulkar of India and Hanif Mohammed of Pakistan became world famous as a teenager. So was the case with one of the greatest footballers of the world, Pele, also known as the Black Pearl, who rose to fame as a teenager.

Very recently, Jannik Sinner, a 22-year-old boy from Italy, won the Singles Championship at Australian Lawn Tennis Championship, in January 2024 and thanked his parents for noticing his talent and supporting his sports career

The similar thing was done my Mr Ajit, the elder brother of Sachin Tendulkar, who noticed Sachin's talent and took 11-year-old Sachin to his Coach Mr Ramakant Achrekar. Both of them contributed immensely to make Sachin Tendulkar, the God of Cricket.

A sportsman's international career lasts for limited years. Hence the people who start early, establish themselves early and can last longer. Parental guidance and support in finding the talent in a child and arranging proper training are extremely important.

Music and Dancing

Bharat Ratna Ms. Lata Mangeshkar, the Melody Queen of India, started professional singing at the age of 13/14. She was learning Indian classical music and   at the same time sang for the movies of Hindi, Marathi, and many other languages as a playback singer.

There are lot of famous professional classical dancers who started learning difficult dance forms from a very young age. Indian classical dances like Bharatanatyam, Kathak, Kathakali, Kuchipudi, etc take many years to master. Pandit Gopi Krishna and Pandit Birju Maharaj were very famous as great Indian classical dancers.

Parents and elders of the family have a huge responsibility in recognizing the talent in a child so that the child can be guided properly to pursue his/her dream career and not be forced to do something following the mass or peers.

As Margaret Mead said, "Children should be taught how to think and not what to think." We should encourage children and students to think, get innovative ideas, and work towards their dream.

A child's psychology and personality change a lot, the moment he steps into 13th year. Being a teenager marks a real change in personal growth. He starts thinking that he is grown-up, his clothing style changes, and he adopts fashionable dress codes. He starts to adopt ways and means to look good and attractive, and at the same time begins to dream about his future. He sees successful and famous people around him and therefore tries to do various things to become a successful person.

At present, there are lot of opportunities as there are many options for professional career. Parents and children have to choose a career which is best for the child and suits the child's interest and passion.

This Decade is thus very important for determining one's career path.

This Decade is also Important for Proper Upbringing of a Child

Character Building

This period is also very important for character building for young ones. The values taught by the parents, teachers, and well-wishers at this stage go a long way. Children are more obedient and more attached at this stage, their personality and future behaviour can, therefore, be molded with love and care and proper attention.

The guidance regarding their studies, mannerism, etiquette, dressing, language, eating habits, general behaviour, respect to elders, and caring for the society must be taught at this stage so that the children understand social behaviour, social norms and eventually, become good human beings, good citizen as well as matured , balanced people , when they grow up.

Developing and adopting good habits at this stage is very important. As most of the parents or single parents work, child care has become very important. Quite often a young child is kept in a creche. A child spends lot of time with helpers or nannies, hence it is important to select the creche, or house helpers, or nannies very carefully. The child will follow these people and be influenced by their habits, language, and values which, in some cases, may not be ideal. Most of the helpers, maids, servants or even nannies are often not educated enough to bring up the child properly. Hence, selection of an educated and well-behaved helper or nanny is very important.

Children, at times, might pick up wrong language, and habits by watching the maids, servants, or even nannies. Some of these helpers may use slang, or may lose temper easily, or get irritated or frustrated, which might be observed by the child and should be avoided as much as possible.

Parents at this stage should try to watch children's area of interest to motivate and guide them to select proper time for studies, keep inspiring them to dream big and help them to work hard to achieve their goal. If the child is studying late at night, parents, either mother or father, can provide a glass of milk, water, or a cup of coffee so that the child can feel that he is not alone and that his parents are supportive and involved as well. He will feel good, motivated, loved and cared for and be more energetic, enthusiastic, and interested in his studies (which at times may seem to be boring and monotonous for him).

Children at this stage want to try out new things. They are under a lot of influence by their peers. The peer pressure might lead them to habits like smoking, drinking, and even doing drugs. They may get into avoidable fights, arguments with other children and may adopt aggressive attitude because of the wrong influence or wrong support of the peers.

Instead, children should be guided and motivated about future goals such as for higher studies, hobbies like music, arts, sports, or other physical activities which are required for a holistic development of a child.

Hobbies

Hobbies are our life-long friends. For instance, a hobby like music can be pursued till 80s or even 90s, which is self-entertaining, satisfying and has lots of positive effect apart from creating friends and getting appreciation for our talents. Hobbies such as reading, writing, painting, sketching, oil painting, or any other creative activities which can be done in our leisure time could be a good hobby. A hobby enables us to spend time in a positive way and it's a nice way to remain engaged.

Albert Einstein was known to play the violin and Piano. Elsa, Einstein's wife, once remarked "I fell in love with Albert because he played Mozart so beautifully on the Violin". Dr. APJ Abdul Kalam, former President of India, used to play Veena, a musical instrument which Devi (Goddess) Saraswati, the Indian Goddess of Education, is seen holding and playing with. Great scientists, philosophers, authors, politicians, leaders pursued some kind of hobby to rejuvenate their energy level. Hobbies keep us happy and positively engaged. It provides us solace; mental comfort and one can spend hours pursuing hobbies. Hobbies are also important in old age, after retirement from the busy professional life, when people have plenty of time. Hobbies save people from boredom. It provides joy, pleasure, energy, and will to survive as it provides great company.

In the old age, when people are neglected and others avoid them and don't talk to them, hobbies provide a positive, meaningful, and entertaining company.

Hobbies, therefore, must be added in a young person's life, depending on his/ her interest, which can be developed alongside the studies and professional career. Adolescence is an ideal stage to pick and progress with the hobbies.

Ages 13/14 to 23/24 is the period when a hobby can be learnt and mastered to make it a lifelong friend. It can also be a career for some who are extremely talented.

How to plan to take fullest advantage of this decider decade.

We have only one life. Those who plan well and work towards attaining their goal, enjoy their lives more. Since parents have the experience of their youth, they can provide guidance in planning the lives and careers of their children.

They can therefore take advantage of their experience and expertise to guide the children.

It is very important to watch carefully our children's interests, and once confirmed, we can plan the progress of a child's development in a planned manner.

If the child is good at maths or accounting and loves the subject, then we must provide proper guidance for him to do even better .He can be motivated to do an MSc or Ph.D. in

Maths or Accounting or a CA, CPA, CFA, MBA (Finance), or Ph.D. in Finance also, to have a good career in professional life.

In a professional career, any line is a good line, provided one excels at it. The world can be harsh, it is 'winner takes it all', so one has to be the best in any line or career he/she chooses. Once the particular language or profession is decided by the child, after proper deliberation and consultation with parents, and teachers, the child should be supported to work hard to learn and achieve mastery on the subject. This decade, from 13/14 to 23/24, is the time to learn, prepare, and work hard to be successful.

The importance of the 'Decider Decade', therefore, must be understood well in advance by the parents to take advantage of this most important decade of our lives.

Super 6 Years

Age 17 to 23 is the most crucial in our career, particularly for our academic career. This is the period when we move to study and get a graduate degree which might be followed by post graduate degree. There are certain post graduate degrees like Master of Business Administration (MBA), etc., where 2 to 4 years of work experience may be required in some countries.

This is the period a student must do his best. A good grade, say first class in graduate degree would enable him/her to get into a good and reputed university for post-graduation.

A good grade in post-graduation like M.Sc. in Supply Chain Management, would open the flood gates of opportunity for a student in job market.

Some students with a good graduation degree, like BSc in Economics, Banking & Finance may like to work for 2 to 4 years and then do MBA from a reputed international university later.

Getting an MBA degree after MSc or Engineering elevates a person's standing to a much higher level as he is considered to be very highly qualified and hence get good International Placement in Good Companies/ Industries. This may happen when a person is in his mid-20s. He would have a long career in his respective field of expertise. Updating skills and increasing relevant qualifications would however, be required to stay ahead of their colleagues and competitors.

It is therefore very important for the parents, teachers, and the students to understand the value of these years, i.e., the years between the age 17 to 23, the super 6 years, of a student's life.

These few years are really vital and can really make a student successful in life so that he does not need to look back in life as he would be one of the most sought-after professional experts in their field.

Importance of super 6 years

Quite often though, students, being young in age do not understand the importance of these few years in their life.

They waste a lot of time exploring wrong things, due to peer pressure, or wrong advice and influence by bad friends or bad company.

As it is the nature of young ones to try out new things, in the stages of growing up, bad friends may pull the good students, both boys and girls into wrong or unwanted things.

This is the period; many growing children of age 17/18 years are drawn to smoking and drinking and even to drugs.

Quite a few students, instead of attending classes in the college, go somewhere else and get involved in unwanted activities, flunking college. They are not only wasting their parent's money but also wasting the golden period of their life when they should work hard, study well, gain knowledge to be successful in life.

Peer pressure during this period of life, i.e., between 17 to 23, plays a very important role in our life and must be monitored properly by the parents to avoid bad peer influence on avoidable things.

Monitoring children for a few important aspects during super 6 years:

Bad Company

There is saying in English, "A man is known by the company he keeps." Quite often, we may meet and make wrong people our friends, being deceived by their sugar quoted talks in the beginning.

Unfortunately, young people without parents or with a single parent are especially vulnerable to falling into such bad company, who may, unfortunately, spoil their lives. These bad people are not only bad company, they also try to drag young ones to parties, picnics and all such places where young ones get easily influenced to go and enjoy. The enjoyment factor, at times, is very interesting and young ones may even make new and interesting friends, who then plan to take them to a few interesting parties, where the young ones learn to enjoy new things, with new friends or company.

All these activities are kept hidden from the parents, bunking classes is a common practice for many students who are either engaged in above mentioned so called interesting activities or even wasting time in college canteen which is known to be a meeting place for many.

Parents, therefore should maintain good interaction with growing children to keep away the bad company. Parent's love, more family celebrations, an enjoyable family atmosphere can keep the growing children at home.

Relationships

Another problem of the young people, i.e., between 17 to 23, is getting into relationships. A relationship, at this age, is actually not properly understood by young ones because very few understand the true meaning of relationship at this stage of life. But many get involved in a bad relationship, especially with opposite sex, and start ignoring studies.

Good students become bad and again parents are unaware of such relationships and wonder how their good children, good students slowly become bad, with deteriorating bad grades in the exams.

In some cases, some of them suffer from mental depression also. They take drugs or even attempt to commit suicide due to unsuccessful relationships.

Parents eventually become aware of these things. But it might be too late to bring back the child's healthy state of mind. Parents, therefore, must interact with the children more at this stage and provide friendly support to keep their children away from wrong company and from any avoidable relationship. Children should be empowered to speak to the parents on any subject without hesitation or fear.

Bad Food Habits

Another very important aspect of super 6 years is, children / growing children at this stage remain busy in studies and other activities but they use cell phone, laptops, tablets, desktops very frequently and when hungry consume all non-consumables like junk food, aerated drinks which make them obese.

The sedentary lifestyle, less physical exercise only adds to the unhealthy lifestyle.

Children, once obese, may struggle to achieve a trim physique, but suffer from inferiority complex in the work place and social circle. They also lose their self-confidence as they do not look good, and cannot wear fashionable dresses any more.

It is therefore very important for the parents to keep a strict watch in the behaviour of the child between 17 to 23 years. Parents should spend more time with the children. Any unusual behaviour must be tackled with patience, politeness, love and maturity. They should also monitor their food habits to keep the children healthy.

Since we know our children best, we must maintain very close relation with them and allow them to speak to us openly, whatever may be the case.

We must try to tell our children about the importance of this period of life. That all the picnics, movies, parties can be enjoyed later on but these golden years from 17 to 23 would never come back. Wasting time during this period, deviating from their life's dream, and goal would only make them average people. And as mediocrity has no place in our life, an average man with basic qualification, might not achieve a higher position in the society.

The age 17 to 23 is probably the most important period of our life, when we must do our best to climb the ladder of success by working hard to achieve our goals in life and establishing us well in the society. The success achieved due to the hard work of these super six years becomes the Harbinger of future Laurels.

Any student who does not understand the value of the period of our age between 17 to 23, the golden period, would miss the bus and would repent throughout his life for ignoring the importance of this, especially the period of the Super Six Years, i.e., the period between 17 years and 23 years, which if properly utilized can really help him become successful in life.

A Humble Request for The Parents

The life of our children, who we love most, is most important. It is my humble request to all parents that we should not push them beyond their limits or else the end result may be very bad. Let the children express their opinion in selecting their career and they would excel in that profession. We should, however, provide all kinds of support to our children needed for their growth and career. It is our duty, with our experience, to spot the talent in a child and guide the child to select a suitable career for himself.

"Free the child's potential and you transform him into the world" –Maria Montessori

CHAPTER V

Skills and Good Practices Required to Keep Life on Track

We have only one life.

Since we have only one life, it cannot be wasted. We have to plan our life to travel the journey well, enjoy it, and achieve the goals planned for and keep the memorable footprints for others to remember and follow in future. This would keep us alive even after we are gone, like for example Great Mahatma Gandhi, Great Abraham Lincoln, Ms. Lata Mangeshkar the great Indian singer, Sir Don Bradman, Cricketer, Albert Einstein the Great Scientist, Rabindranath Tagore the Great poet, William Shakespeare the Great writer etc.

Dream big to shape your life.

We have to dream big to achieve something spectacular to become successful in life. If we dream big, we will start working for it, prepare hard to achieve our goals, while those of us who do not dream big or not dream at all to do well in life, lead a mediocre life and struggle throughout life, remaining merely a passenger. The near and dear ones including family, and even parents also suffer because of the lackadaisical attitude, of such people, towards life.

As Dr. APJ Abdul Kalam, the former President of India, said "Dream is not that you see in sleep, dream is something that does not let you sleep." Hence our dream determines our will to succeed. We must, therefore, dream big and shape our life to become successful and make people around us happy.

CASE STUDY--1 : Seeing a Big Dream

Sudhir Dholakia (Name changed), a young man came to Bombay(now Mumbai), in early 60s. He started working with a Builder, owner of a Building Construction Company. Bombay was becoming a popular destination for many people as it was turning into the Financial Capital of India. The demand for housing was going up.

Sudhir saw the successful builder and was highly inspired by him. He had a Big Dream of becoming a Big Builder one day.

He worked for a few years with the builder. He then wanted to complete his education.

He got admission in an Engineering College to study B.Tech in Civil Engineering.

On a Sunday, he went on a picnic with his friends to a remote place called Mira Road East. The railway line, which connected Bombay with Gujarat and beyond, passed through Mira Road, a small Railway Station. The eastern side of the railway line was known as Mira Road East and the western side was Mira Road west, which was totally

Marshy Area, being very close to the sea. There were very few small huts and few small buildings in Mira Road East. The area was vast, partly marshy and sparsely populated. A narrow road connected Mira Road with Bhayandar, a bigger place than Mira Road.

Mira Road was located next to Dahisar, where Greater Bombay Municipality limit ended. An undeveloped area but close to the Greater Mumbai Municipal Area.

Sudhir decided to buy some land at Mira Road East, which was partly Marshy but very cheap as no one wanted to go to such a remote area. Sudhir, however thought that, as Bombay was growing, Mira Road, being so close to Greater Bombay, would also grow eventually.

For a few years he kept the land unused and concentrated on his work with the same Builder even after he completed his B.Tech and gained valuable experience in building construction.

Indian economy saw a big change in 1991 and the economy opened up and started doing well.

In early 90s there was a Real Estate Boom in Mumbai (name of Bombay became Mumbai) and Mira Road Land started becoming costly. Suddenly a lot of Builders wanted to make Residential Buildings in Mira Road East because of the high cost in main Mumbai and heavy demand in Mira Road.

Sudhir started his Building Construction Company in January,1992 and named it as Dholakia Constructions Ltd. He hired Civil Engineers, Architects and launched his first project, a 10 storied, Residential Apartment Building in Mira Road East, using part of his land.

The project was a great success, as it was completed on time, flats were sold in record time as good publicity was done and the local Real Estate Agents were taken into confidence. The project was liked by the customers because of the good quality of the construction as well as the good quality Amenities.

Sudhir did not look back since then. He had huge land at his disposal, bought long back, at a very cheap rate, he had vast experience in building constructions and was aware of customer's choice. Dholakia Constructions became a Famous Builder in Mumbai, and now has it's Projects in every part of Mumbai.

Sudhir thus became a big and reputed builder and accomplished his Big Dream.

Q1. What was Sudhir's, a poor man's big dream?

Q2. How his business acumen accrued immense benefits in future?

Q3. How did Sudhir accomplish his dream?

Ans of Q1.

Working in a Building Construction Company, gave Sudhir an idea of becoming a builder one day. The success of the Builder, Inspired him to become a famous builder in future.

Ans of Q2.

Sudhir, while working with the builder, developed good Business Acumen. He dreamt of becoming a famous builder one day and for that, he realised that he had to do the following things:

a) Buy a piece of land at a cheap rate, at a place which had great potential to become a popular Residential Destination in future.

b) He should buy at a rate he could afford and at a place, which was not a priority for others.

c) He understood that Housing would become a big business in Bombay (now Mumbai) as it was fast becoming a Popular Destination for many. He should plan to become a Builder in future.

d) He should buy the land as early as possible, though undeveloped and unpopular now but with huge potential of growth in future.

His business acumen, of anticipating the development of business in future, made him successful.

Ans of Q3.

Sudhir prepared himself to fulfil his dream. He took following steps:

a) Learnt the skills of building construction, learning the minute details.
b) Acquired the qualification of B.Tech in Civil Engineering
c) Hired experienced Civil Engineers and Architects

d) He started his own Building Construction Company at an appropriate time in 1992 when Indian Economy opened up and the business was growing and Indian Economy started doing well. He gave lot of importance to Quality of Building Construction, Amenities and facilities, which made Dholakia Constructions very popular and reliable builder.

e) Adopted apt measures for Marketing the Flats of his building and sold the flats very fast to get back the capital quickly, which could be used for the new projects.

As the demand of Residential Properties increased in Mira Road East, Sudhir became a famous builder very soon, because he saw A Big Dream and worked hard to accomplish it. His vision, meticulous planning, timely execution made his dream, A Great Success.

Educate your Mind and Heart, both.

"Educating the mind without educating the heart is no education at all" – Aristotle

It is extremely important that we educate our mind and heart both. Only then we will be able to respect people, tolerate people, and love people irrespective of their cast, creed, religion, region, colour, culture, language etc.

This quality is extremely important to become a good citizen internationally. The globalization needs international approach, mindset, attitude and liberal as well as broad minded nature. Educating mind and heart would help us achieve that. It avoids all kind of discrimination, promotes brotherhood and helps in achieving spirituality.

Some important skills for a Hassle -Free Life

Avoid Shortcuts in life

It's part of human nature to seek shortcuts. We take short cuts to save time, to get quick success, to impress others, to manipulate our financial state, to overtake our colleagues in professional life and so on, but invariably the so-called shortcuts lead us to a more complicated as well as longer journey.

For example, let's say a man with his girlfriend is trying to reach the movie theatre fast, is driving his car fast and jumps the traffic signal and unfortunately gets caught by the traffic police, he would then have to spend 10 to 15 extra minutes dealing with the police instead of waiting at the traffic signal for ½ minute or pay penalty as well as face embarrassment for this act, being caught on the Camera. So shortcut usually ends up being a costlier experience hence should be avoided.

Similarly, a business man adopting malpractices in business to get rich faster may get in to a lot of problem when checked and caught by the regulatory bodies, hence avoidable.

It is therefore very important to teach children to avoid any kind of shortcuts in life, which ultimately saves time, money, earns respect, and preserves a person's dignity.

Have Self-control

We must learn to have self-control. The power of self-control saves us from a lot of avoidable problems and teaches us to regulate our habits, nature, behaviour, life style, and language which makes a person balanced and acceptable in civilized society.

It is important to have control over the following:

Shed Ego

We must control or learn to manage our ego. Ego is the biggest enemy of a person. It gives a sense of false supremacy to the person which may spoil a well-established relationship. One may repent later on but the damage is already done due to this so-called ego.

There is a lot of difference between self-pride, self-confidence and ego. Self-pride and self-confidence allow a person to live with dignity and perform better but ego is based on a false sense of superiority that may not be acceptable to others including close friends, relatives, and even near and dear ones. Ego is harmful, always has negative effects, and must be avoided.

Win over your Mood

Mood is the way a person feels at a particular time. He/she may feel happy or unhappy. If happy, he/she would behave in a positive way, and if unhappy, he/she wouldn't talk to friends, and may not be willing to keep their request. For example, in a friendly get together, friends request another friend to sing a song for them but if the person is not in the mood, he/she will not meet the request of his/her friends. He/she will keep to himself/herself and may not even speak to the friends for some time. Mood, therefore, must be controlled or managed well otherwise it will make a person indifferent which is an unwanted quality of a good person. People even friends avoid such people.

Never lose your Temper:

Temper is the expression of our anger. All of us, at times, get angry for something which has not happened as we desired. A child gets angry if he is not given a chocolate he wants, a child may be angry if he does not get the ball he wants, a student gets angry if he has performed badly in an exam that he otherwise knew well, a person may get angry if he cannot crack a job interview, a lover may be angry if his girlfriend does not show up on time and so on. When angry, we tend to lose our temper which may or may not be justified. With practice we begin to learn to manage our temper and lead a very happy and pleasant life. There are lot of things which can be managed without losing our temper. For example, your wife while making a cup of tea in the early morning forgets to add sugar for you (if you are used to sugar), you get angry and utter some harsh or unpleasant words right in the morning and spoil the day. Instead, keep quiet for some time, the moment she would take a sip of tea she would realize that the sugar was missing, or just politely tell it to her because everybody makes a mistake. She would go quickly to get sugar for both of you. A little wait and patience would make the day a pleasant one, on the contrary your anger would have spoilt the day and would have made you ungrateful for the endeavour your wife made to make a cup of tea, early in the morning.

Another common example could be, you are in theatre to watch a new movie and some arguments take place between your girlfriend and some strangers and you also join your girlfriend in the heated argument. Both parties losing temper, make the situation ugly and terrible, instead you can try to solve the issue by shifting your girlfriend away from the scene, and avoiding arguments. Because you went there to enjoy the evening with your girlfriend, see the movie and not spoil the evening by getting into avoidable arguments.

If the situation does not improve due to the arrogance of the other party, then involve the other viewers or multiplex staff/security to resolve the issue in an amicable and matured manner, keeping in view the safety and security as well as respect of your girlfriend and yourself.

Develop Positive Attitude

It is the way in which a person views and evaluates something or someone, a predisposition or a tendency to respond positively or negatively towards a certain idea, object, person or situation.

There are 4 types of Attitude:-

1. Positive Attitude:

Positive attitude is a positive mindset of a person. A positive person is always in a happy state of mind, accepts good and bad things in a positive way. He is optimistic, treats the world in a fair way. A very mature, loving, caring, helpful person, who accepts things as they come, smilingly.

2. Negative Attitude

People with negative attitude are unhappy, as they have a negative mindset. They doubt everything and do not trust people. They are frustrated, disgruntled and uncertain. They spoil the environment wherever they are, they usually have no friends.

3. Neutral Attitude

These people are indifferent, non-committal and try to remain neutral. They are well-balanced in life and remain with a neutral approach. They are complacent and self-satisfied. They neither help nor take any help, the silent and secluded lot in the society. They remain detached and therefore have very few friends. They are quite often boring, monotonous and unenthusiastic.

4. Sickken Attitude.

This attitude is the combination of negativity and aggressiveness. They make people around them feel sick with their very uncommon and aggressive attitude, no one likes them. They are unfit in any organization as they cannot be a team player. They consider that everything is bad in this world and only they are right.

We should therefore try to adopt Positive Attitude which would help us in our personal and professional life.

Adopt Good Habits

Habit is a behaviour that is repeated frequently. This kind of behaviour can be an action, a routine or a lifestyle.

Habits can be of following types:

- Good Habits – Getting up early in the morning every day, exercising daily, thinking positively and following win-win policy.
- Bad Habits – Excessive Smoking, excessive drinking, negative thinking, procrastination, nail-biting, etc.

Habits shapes a person's personality. A man with good habits is respected in the society, his habits, behaviour, language, and attire make him a gentleman. People get attracted towards him, become friends, well-wishers, and companions. He is accepted in the work place, in social circle as he is liked by people for his habits and behaviour. On the other hand, a person with bad habits is repulsive, and avoided by people. He is not easily accepted in work place and social circle as he exhibits bad habits like excessive smoking, excessive drinking, using foul language, getting angry, aggressive nature, and improper attire, etc.

Learn to Manage Your Emotion

Emotion is a short-lived feeling that comes from a known cause. It can make us happy or sad or angry or dejected because of this known cause. This cause could make us smile or cry. For example, a student getting the news that he has topped the class in the exam becomes very happy and may even jump in joy. A man losing money in the race course becomes sad. One can become emotional by seeing a close friend's misery, more so if he is unable to help his friend.

Emotion is a mental state which changes as per the situation as explained above. It has a temporary effect on us. One should be emotionally balanced, and strong to deal with the various causes that may affect our mind and brain, in a positive way or matured way, so that any news, good or bad, does not affect us mentally or physically, and we do not react by exhibiting an emotional outburst, which may lead to more harm to our mental state as well as body.

There are, however, situations and incidents which may cause emotional breakdown and these are the situations which are extremely difficult to handle. We have to learn to be mentally strong to handle such situations, particularly to help others, needing our help.

Quite often we hear young ones tragically committing suicide because of a failed relationship or getting terribly depressed because of failing in an exam or job interview. We must, therefore, learn to control our emotion so that we can avoid getting affected by the various causes / issues that could sway our emotional balance.

We have to learn to be strong to survive in this uncertain and, at times, harsh world. We should learn to face the difficulties as a part of our complex journey of life.

We should remember what Dr APJ Abdul Kalam had once said, "Man needs difficulties in life because these are necessary to enjoy success".

Emotional Quotient (EQ)

Emotional Quotient is the most important quality of an employee in any organization at present. Every organization needs an emotionally balanced, stable and emotionally mature individual to run the organization.

A man's behaviour, from morning to evening, should be constant. May it be a shop floor, corporate office or football field or a boxing ring, control over emotion and emotional balance makes a person perform better.

Control your Mind

The mind is a person's set of intellectual or mental facilities. It refers to the group of cognitive psychiatric process that includes facilities like perception, memory, reasoning, thinking, desire, emotion, sensation etc.

Our brain controls our mind, but it's difficult because our mind is restless, super-fast, imaginative, very light to move around, very emotional, sentimental, a great thinker and always out of grasp.

Brain tries very hard to control the mind and time and again tries to bring it back from floating around in the air. Mind, in my opinion, has three sides:

- Positive – With positive and constructive thoughts.

- Negative – With negative, unpleasant even evil thoughts at times.
- Dormant / Inert – While sleeping the mind is inert, it is not active and not thinking about anything.

Since our mind is a limitless, wild, and imaginative phenomenon, it is extremely important to learn to control our mind.

We have to learn to keep our mind:

- Positive
- Innovative
- Constructive
- Keep the mind enclosed in our body, brain and soul so that it does not float in the imaginative or abstract world, in continuous wilderness, not allowing the person to work or concentrate on work, which the person wants to peruse.

We have to learn to keep our mind in a positive, constructive, and planned path or else the time will be wasted doing nothing. Mind should be controlled to get better results, while uncontrolled mind with idle brain can cause a lot of trouble in our domestic as well as professional life. Mind is the most precious possession of a human being and must be nurtured, controlled, and guided by our brain for own benefit.

Positive Mind

Our mind is restless, fast moving and can think positive things, negative things, absurd things, destructive / offensive things. We are all normal human beings. We are not saints, but with our good upbringing, good education and maturity we must learn to control the thought process of our mind. We must guide our mind to think positive things. Positiveness keeps us happier and peaceful. Negative thoughts are harmful, and hence must be avoided. A person with positive thoughts and positive mindset can concentrate better on:

- His studies
- His work
- Doing good things
- Being creative and innovative
- Being helpful to own family as well as the society
- Being liked by everyone

Innovative Mind

People with innovative mind are the real assets of the society. They help the society with their innovative ideas. They are the people who help the mankind by their inventions and discoveries. E.g., Einstein, James Watt, Newton, Steve Jobs, and many more.

Their innovative mind always wanted to do something different, to think out of the box, to help the people and the society. It is their innovative mindset that made them work hard and sacrifice their youth, their life to help the mankind.

And now, they have become immortal because of their valuable contribution to the society.

Creative Mind

Like innovative mind, people with creative mindset are also assets of the society. People with creative mindset always create something good for the people and the society. The poets, the writers, the artists, and the musicians have always helped the society.

Great people like Shakespeare, George Bernard Shaw, Rabindranath Tagore, Leonardo Da Vinci, Mozart, and Beethoven are famous even today because of their great creations.

If we learn to control and guide our mind to be creative, we can achieve numerous things.

On the other hand, there are people who harbor sheltered negative / destructive ideas in their minds and become anti-social elements, and criminals. These kind of people spoil their life, the only life they have.

Meditation and Spirituality can be very useful in controlling and guiding our restless as well as uncontrollable mind.

Some Suggestions to Improve our life

Learn to Adjust

We must learn to adopt one of the best qualities and that is the quality to adjust.

The world works as per its own requirements and the people behave as per their own habits, needs, and circumstances as well. It is different than how we want them to behave. As we also don't behave as they want us to behave. But we have to survive in this world, with its people. Every set-up is different, there are social norms, and official laws which have to be adhered to, to live in the society. It may be the school football team, our married life, the office in which we are working, everywhere we will have to learn to adjust and accommodate other's behaviour, norms, and laws, etc., which is known as adjustment.

We may like to sleep late in the morning but to reach school, college, or even office we will have to get up early so that we are not late. In a group of friends, we may have to accommodate the desire of others to enjoy the moment and forcing own wish may spoil the fun. We will have to learn to adjust to remain friendly with our friends, we will have to adjust with our spouse, who'll come from a different family, or even different culture, and we will have to adjust in our work place, to become a good team member and an acceptable working executive.

The power of adjustment enables us to be mentally happy as the power or technique of adjustment automatically removes all elements of tension, may it be in a school classroom, or on a road while driving, or in an office where others, who are equally smart, qualified and experienced, are working along with us.

The quality of adjustment plays an extremely important role in our domestic, personal, as well as professional life. A person who can adjust is always happy.

Failure or Rejections is a part of our life.

"It is fine to celebrate success, but it is more important to head the lessons of failure" – Bill Gates

Failure and rejection are normal experiences of our life. "A person who never made a mistake never tried anything new" – Albert Einstein.

So, failure is unavoidable if we are doing something new like trying to work on new innovation, discovery or trying to learn something. While learning cycling, we fall many times and it happens with everybody, but that is how we learn because every time we fall, we learn the trick of cycling and eventually become successful.

Failure teaches us to prepare hard and better which leads us to our success eventually. Every failure teaches us a lot of things, which enables us to succeed in future.

Take the example of Wright Brothers who invented Aeroplane. They failed countless times in their experiments and then finally succeeded on an almost impressible mission. Today, the entire world is enjoying on their hard-earned success.

People had only heard or read about the Flying Chariot in Indian religious epic, 'Ramayana', used by Ravan, the king of Lanka, and always thought it was Saint Valmiki, the writer of Ramayana's, wild imagination.

Wright Brothers, in addition to their extremely difficult project, faced a lot of criticism while convincing the world about the possibility of their success that one day people would be able to fly in an aeroplane like a Flying Chariot. Their multiple failures did not deter them or demotivate them.

Like failure, rejections are also part of our life. Quite often people reject our idea. Rejection is very common for a Marketing, or Sales professional, as convincing people to buy a new product is a difficult task. But a sales person has to survive, hence learning to negotiate and win over rejection is his top priority. Like failure, rejection also teaches us a lot of things like patience, improving the skills of logic, convincing the customer. Rejection must not demotivate us but should encourage us to master the skills of converting rejection into acceptance.

It is a wonderful life but bad habits can spoil it, choice is yours

We live on planet Earth. The only planet known to us, where human beings are living and it is beautiful. It has hills, trees, plants, flowers, fruits, rivers, seas, snow, deserts, enough water to drink, oxygen to breath, and sunlight to look after all of us including plants.

The modern technology has made life extremely easy, enjoyable, and happy. In fact, mankind was never happier before. The life span is also increasing with the gift of advanced medical science. Japan, already has a club where people more than 100 years of age, are members of '100 years club'.

But this wonderful life is dependent on us, our habits, and our way of life. God has given us everything in terms of resources of the world. Our parents give us everything to make sure we're comfortable and happy, but as we grow-up, we get influenced by our peers and outside world, we adopt new habits like smoking, drinking, eating junk food etc. Some people even get into the company of people taking drugs.

All these habits are extremely bad for our health. Our body cannot digest all these items. Take for example of our intestine which is located inside our stomach, it is a single celled pipe and cannot take the burden of excessive liquor / hard drinks. The same goes for our liver and kidneys, they get burdened by all the wrong intake inside the body and results in people getting various diseases and our life gets ruined. A person who could live 100 years ends up dying in 40s and 50s, or even earlier at times.

So, it is extremely important to understand and realise that living a longer and healthy life is in our own hand . God has given us a wonderful life, parents make it comfortable, but we may spoil it with our bad and avoidable habits. Our life does not belong to us only, it also belongs to our parents, family and the society we live in. We have to look after our parents in their old age, and the society as it is our responsibility and we cannot ruin our life with bad habits. The so-called 'enjoyment' should be within limits in order to have longer enjoyable life.

Try to become a Skilful Specialist

This is the era of specialization. One has to be a specialist and excel in his field. Quite often we think about unemployment which has become prevalent in almost all countries of the world. A skilled person, however, would always get a job somehow because of his skills and someone, or some organization can utilize it.

Once I had approached the General Manager (GM) of a company for a job of one of my known persons. Since I knew the GM, a job was offered to my man, but the salary was very low. I almost jokingly, since I knew him, told him that my personal driver gets more than this and this person is much more educated than my driver, hence his salary should be higher. The GM replied 'Your driver is a skilled person, and because of him you can relax in your car but this person is a fresh university graduate, I will have to train him for some time until he becomes useful to my organization.'

Being skilful therefore is very important and there is no dearth of jobs for a skilled person.

We must therefore explain to our children whether they decide to become a Doctor, or an Engineer, or a Chartered Accountant, or an Artist, or a sportsperson that they have to become a specialist in their field so that people would consider them an expert and look, and search for them.

Employment will come to them, that is the importance of being skilful. But a skilful person has to constantly work hard to remain ahead of other competitors within his field, by acquiring new qualifications, and training and keeping themselves constantly updated.

A Moment's Happiness Gained from a Wrong/Avoidable Source Can Ruin Our Life

During our youth, we want to try out different things. As we grow-up, we leave behind certain things as we consider them harmful, but a few of us are quite careless about our own lives.

Our lives are safer as long as we are in the custody of our parents, but when we go to a hostel or abroad for higher studies, we live on our own. Our style of living, habits, and peer pressure become very important in our lives. Quite often, we indulge in things that are harmful and dangerous.

Especially when we go to another station or abroad to work, we remain away from our parents and, if married, from our families at times. We spend leisure time alone, or with some friends. It is extremely important to keep good friends and be in their company. Bad friends with bad habits, or an erratic lifestyle will pull us to do wrong things or things we are not used to doing or do not want to do. E.g., spending late nights in a pub, getting into drugs, or getting the habit of having sex with just anyone, even strangers. All these habits can give us temporary happiness, but they can ruin our life in the long run. We must be smart enough to ensure safety and security of ourselves. A moment's mistake, with the influence of wrong friends, is enough to spoil our life. Our hard work, good education, high academic degrees, parent's dream, and our own dreams will all vanish if we get a bad disease like Cancer, AIDs, and liver cirrhosis etc, due to drugs, or excessive drinking or excessive smoking.

Life is a marathon; we have to run along with it, keeping ourselves safe, secure, healthy, and happy. Our lives revolve around many other lives, such as those of our families, children, and parents. Therefore, we must be smart, mature, careful, and responsible. A simple lifestyle, living within limits would be helpful in the long run. One should aim to enjoy life throughout, not just for one night.

Select a Career with the Help of Your Parents and Teachers and Work Towards It.

The professional life, in our life, plays a major role, It normally starts around the age of 20s and goes till 70s and even beyond for some people. Professional life dictates progress in our life. It gives us money, status, respect, standing in our society. A person with good profession is automatically respected in the society, e.g. a doctor. A person, who is a doctor by profession, is highly respected person in the society, and throughout the world because it is a noble profession. Doctors are always helpful to the people of the society and aid those who are helpless. Doctors are almost like a 'Demi Gods' to all of us. They deal with the very existence, the life, of a person. Their treatment and medicine can save lives.

Since profession in a man's life is so important, it is extremely important to spot the talent in a child, try to discuss his area of interest and pursue his/her career after selecting the career very carefully by the parents, and teachers, and child himself. Once decided, based on the talent, area of interest, and capability, one has to plan and work hard to become an excellent professional. One has to try and work hard to become an excellent professional in one's field.

The world is a tough battle field and only the best can survive. We have to, therefore, follow what Aristotle had once said, "Excellence then, is a habit, and not an accident."

We have to adopt the habit of performing with excellence, to be one of the best in the field.

It is therefore very important to select proper profession and then learn to excel in the profession to become successful in our life.

Be open to Re-Skilling and New Opportunities

New skills are emerging in the world. The advancement in technology, the changing lifestyle, the modern world with digitized and globalized business, needs new skills. The skills have been changing in past also, as seen during industrial revolution in IR-I , in 18th Century, which introduced steam power, IR-II in 19th Century, which gave electricity and mass production. Power loom replaced handlooms. IR-III,in 20th Century, which gave us computers, internet and clerks lost their jobs. At present, it is the era of Artificial Intelligence now, and IR-IV is taking place. Robots and Cranes are replacing labour force in the factories, building construction industry. Advanced technology has precision work, greater quality and discovering new area of business and operations. Cars will be driver-less, planes and drones will be unmanned, robots will reduce the use of manpower, block chain, and machine learning will be more useful and economical. Hence, old skills may not get us any jobs in the coming future. Car drivers will have to learn new skills to survive, labours will have to learn new skills to survive, and all of us will have to learn new skills to survive in the work place. The new opportunities must be seen and understood. We must take advantage of new opportunities to take benefit from. New subjects must be added in school and college syllabus, new skills must be taught in the engineering colleges, and in all professional colleges like, medicine, management, etc., to educate the professionals with up-to-date knowledge and new skills.

We should therefore attend new courses, get qualifications on the latest subjects, and re-skill ourselves to remain relevant and employable, in addition to our basic qualifications.

Accept Change, It is Inevitable

Change is inevitable in this world. The modern lifestyle, the advanced technology, improved communication systems, improved mobility, frequent discoveries and innovations emerging of IR-IV the Artificial Intelligence, all these things together, are changing the world at a very fast pace.

The consumer behaviour and demand are constantly changing, the working in the offices, factories, and business environment are changing. The jobs, required skills, qualifications required for the jobs, are changing.

The globalization, the trend of urbanization, the changing trend of dressing, eating habits, and transportation are all very evident. We all are seeing the change taking place in every sphere of our life.

We therefore must prepare ourselves for the changing time, changed requirements to be 'in the swim' properly or else we will be left out.

Lack of computer knowledge is no more an excuse. Subjects like AI (Artificial Intelligence), Robotics, Block Chain, machine learning, new language like Python etc., must be learnt and mastered to remain relevant in our work place, social life, even in our domestic life.

It is very important to change our mindset for adopting change in every sphere of our life, may it be personal, domestic or professional.

Modern trends, new technologies, and new techniques must be learnt to survive in modern times. We must therefore adopt changes willingly and faster, to remain ahead of others to become successful in our life.

Since change is a constant phenomenon, we must be mentally ready to act accordingly to adopt the changes to continue being useful to the society.

CHAPTER VI

Some Good Qualities Required to become Successful

Communication Skills

Communication skills play a very crucial part in our lives. The globe has now become a village, it is the communication skills which enable us to speak to our friends, parents, office colleges, and authorities all over the globe. Even global job interviews are now done on telephones. Communication skills, therefore, have become very important now. We all know that communication is a two-way procedure. The most important aspect is that both the parties should understand what the other person is trying to communicate.

Communication skills are of the following types: -

a) Verbal Communication - Verbal Communication is incredibly important as it helps us how we speak, with our language, and vocabulary. We must ensure that the person we are speaking to understands us clearly. Verbal communication in fact is one of the most effective form of communication. We can communicate much more in less time as well as clarify any doubt almost instantly at the spot.

b) Written Communication - Written Communication also plays a very important part in expressing ourselves. The content of expression is in writing. It is a written document; hence, language, expression, and content must be clear, concise, and legally correct as it can also serve as an evidence in future. Written communication is permanent in nature and hence must be properly written. The correct grammar, decent language and right expression are important and the language should be polite and proper. The Emails, WhatsApp, Messages must be written very carefully and properly.

c) Non-verbal communication (body language) - Non-verbal communication is the oldest type of communication, used from ancient times. It also serves a very important role, as all of us use non-verbal communication or body language in our daily lives. It should be used properly with decent and acceptable body language norms. Body language is, at times, also used as code language if we do not want others to understand our communication, and is used in sports quite often. One of the popular body language is the sign of 'thumbs up' or 'V' for victory.

Soft Skills

It is the personal attribute that enables someone to interact effectively and harmoniously with other people.

Soft skills are extremely important to survive in the present era, soft skills include:

- Communication- It is a two-way method to understand each other. Simple words, decent language, good respectful expression is important, as explained earlier.
- Leadership
- Problem Solving
- Emotional, intelligence
- Adaptability
- Team Work
- Decision Making

- Social Skills
- Patience
- Confidence
- Empathy
- Flexibility
- Good Etiquette
- Mannerism
- Decent Behaviour

Soft skills are extremely important to succeed in personal as well as professional life in today's time.

Sincerity

Sincerity is a quality in a person which everyone appreciates. One is expected to be sincere and committed in personal, domestic, and professional life. It is a quality which promotes friendship, earns respect of people, and enormous success. Since everyone likes a sincere and committed person, he becomes the most sought-after person in the society and in any organization.

A non-sincere person is not liked by anyone as he cannot be trusted. He is typically known to be fake or phony and he cannot be given any task or any responsibility as he cannot be trusted.

A non-sincere person is therefore an unpopular, neglected person in the society who is not well-liked by anyone.

Sincerity is therefore an essential quality which must be maintained at all times, in every walk of life. It is extremely important quality to become successful in life.

Integrity

Integrity or honesty is one of the most crucial qualities of a person. This is a quality which can make or break a person, his life, and his career. Everyone is expected to be honest in his behaviour, in his dealings, in his day to day business.

If by any chance, one is found to be dishonest then people usually start avoiding him. No one would then trust him and he won't be welcome anywhere.

No one wants a dishonest man in his company or organization as he cannot be trusted.

In the recent years, there have been cases of insider trading, misappropriation of organization's wealth for own benefit, etc., by very senior professionals. Even some well-known companies/organizations were found to be involved in dishonest practices and they simply vanished from the market.

Today, almost every industry/business has gone international and no one would be willing tolerate a person or an organization without honesty and integrity.

Resilience

Our life is not a bed of roses. Life is tough and it has ups and downs. It includes success and failures, good times and bad times, but we have to sail through this uncertain, unpredictable, and complex journey of life. Quite often, things happen which are not planned. Things do not take place as planned. All of us go through the uncertainty of circumstances including health and our well-being.

We must try to learn to be resilient so that we can stand up after every failure, we can turn around bad time into good time, and convert failure into success.

Resilience teaches us to be tough and gives the strength to fight back, and face this unpredictable world properly.

After all it is our life and we must succeed to be happy in our life and make our parents and other family members happy. We must therefore need to learn to be resilient which is an extremely valuable quality to be successful in our life.

Team Spirit

"If you want to go fast, go alone, but if you want to go far, go along with others." In modern world we must be a team player. Collaboration is extremely vital for any success. We all are inter-dependent on others. Co-operation, collaboration, helping each other, and utilizing each other's expertise enhances team's performance, and organization's performance.

In today's world of globalization and digitization, we work in small teams in various parts of the world. We must understand the method of team building, ethos of team spirit to become a proper team person.

The entire team must have trust and confidence in us when we work as a member of a team.

Sincerity, loyalty, commitment, up-to-date knowledge, and expertise are very important to become and remain an important team member. We must therefore, learn what is team spirit, to remain a relevant team member.

Updating knowledge

In this ever-changing world, where technology is changing very fast, the industry practices are changing, knowledge bases are changing, lifestyle is changing, consumer behaviour is changing, climatic conditions are changing, world order is changing, business and economy are subjected to VUCA, i.e., volatility, uncertainty, complexity, and ambiguity (and even chaotic at times), updating our knowledge to remain relevant in this world is extremely important.

The world's political scenario, availability of basic resources e.g. oil, gas, food, power, etc., the changing economic scenario, the global supply chain problems, emergence of new political, military and economic alliances, are changing the global business and political environment constantly.

The emergence of IR-4, the Artificial Intelligence is also changing the world in big way.

Updating knowledge has become extremely important to survive in the world.

To be Tech Savvy

The Earth is approx. 2.4-billion-year-old and human civilization is more than 600-million-year-old.

But the world started changing from the 18th century as the first Industrial Revolution came with invention of steam power by Thomas Saver, Thomas Newcomen and James Watt.

We are now in the era of IR-4 because of the emergence of Artificial Intelligence, which is again changing the world, leading us to the world of Metaverse, robotics, block chain. IR-4 is promoting machine learning, and much more. The new technologies are emerging every day to bring in changes in every part of our life.

Clerks have been replaced by computers, labourers in the factories have been replaced by robots, drivers are being replaced by driverless cars, drones, un-manned aircrafts, and underwater vessels are without pilots, now. Even Start-Up offices are functioning from Starbucks and other eateries, initially, to save cost of office space. Work From Home

Concept is also the new norm for many Start -Ups and even many established business houses.. The world is really changing fast.

We all have to learn and adopt new skills, learn new technology, and become tech savvy to learn fast changing technologies to remain relevant in this world or else we will perish.

We have to improve our mindset to be alert, active and fast learners of changing technologies to survive in this fast-changing world. We must learn to be tech-savvy to remain relevant in this world.

Accepting Additional Responsibilities

Accepting additional responsibilities is a unique quality of a person which enhances his image in the organization and even in the society.

Every one works as per his area of responsibilities in an organization. His bosses monitor this and his salary and promotion depend on that.

But when a person is given additional responsibilities or one accepts additional responsibilities, he is considered more efficient, competent and trustworthy. These are the people, who are considered to have potential to move up in the ladder of the organization. In our society, people who accepts additional responsibilities, are highly respected and people approach them for consultation, help, and advice.

A man needs to have a big heart, guts, competence, and willpower to accept additional responsibilities.

These kinds of people form a very small percentage in any organization and also in the society.

They are invariably the leaders of the society.

Maintaining Own Dignity

One of the most important qualities of a person is to maintain own self-respect and dignity. It is understood that a person needs to be amicable, balanced, matured, friendly, sober, and respectful. We also grow up in a diverse environment, as most of us study in our own country and abroad, in different culture, environment, climatic conditions, etc. We meet various type of people as our colleagues, bosses, mentors, etc.

At times, under peer pressure, we may adopt different lifestyle, culture, eating habits, sacrificing, at times, even values we learnt from our parents/teachers during our childhood.

Be it as it may, we must at all times, safeguard our self-respect and dignity. Dignity must not be compromised.

Dignity, once compromised, our moral goal post of the life will keep shifting and that may lead us to unlimited problems, because we have now started giving in to demands of people, which may not only be unjust but also harmful.

Fox example, some people have a habit of visiting pubs after office hours and spend a lot of time there socializing, drinking, smoking, dancing, even with strangers.

It is an accepted norm that youngsters follow in most part of the world. Going to pub is one thing but excessive drinking over long hours and adopting habits like smoking, which is injurious to health, since few others are doing, or even getting into some other habits which may make our life more complicated, where keeping our own dignity becomes difficult as we may lose control under the influence of excessive drinking, must be avoided. Some friends may indulge in some activities, where our values may have to be compromised, and other friends may not mind it. We must take a call whether to sacrifice our own culture and values to satisfy our friends, colleagues, or even bosses or should we maintain our values and keep our dignity. As our work place, residence, and friends would keep changing every few years in the global working condition, and we cannot keep changing our values as per demands of our new friends and colleagues. Sycophancy must be avoided. Any circumstances where we tend to forget the value of our self-respect and dignity must be avoided, as,

"A Man Without Dignity, is the Poorest Man of the World."

Sober Habits

A man is known by his habits. A person who speaks too much, is too loud and aggressive, smokes too much, drinks too much, picks up a fight every now and then, loses his temper very often, is egoistic, feels he is greater than everyone else is not liked by people. In fact, people avoid him, he will be a misfit in a team or people won't work with him in a team.

Such people cannot survive in any organization or in any relationship. It is, therefore, very important for all of us to note that the world does not like our individual whims and fancies, but we have to conform to the people's requirements to exist in this world and that is only possible if we inculcate sober habits like speaking softly, have manners and etiquettes, balanced behaviour with amicable approach towards the world. We must understand that people and the organizations have to accept us as friends and colleagues or else we will be left alone.

Sober habits are habits which enable a man to speak softly, makes him balanced, well-behaved, and pleasant. Sober habits make a man likeable, loved, and acceptable in the society.

Doing right things and following right examples.

We have only one life. There is no time to waste. Intelligent and smart people understand that. Life also does not give many opportunities. We must therefore try to inculcate the habit of doing right things, involve in doing proper activities, maintaining the correct direction of progress.

We should also follow right people and the right examples set by them so that we can follow them and learn to be successful like them following their foot-steps.

On the contrary, if we follow wrong people or wrong examples, we may spoil our lives.

There are a lot of examples in society around us of people who are failures. They lead an erratic lifestyle, follow unethical methods, and have improper values.

E.g., people who get involved in gambling, excessive drinking, smoking, are into drugs, making money in illegal and unethical ways, getting involved in anti-social activities, smuggling, and other improper, illegal, or avoidable acts, spoil their lives and those of their families, as well as their loved ones. No one is happy to be related to them, no one is proud of them. They just exist as parasites of the society and as a social burden.

Instead, if we follow the people like Warren Buffet, Bill Gates, Azim Premji, Mother Teresa, Florence Nightingale, etc., we would help the society and its people and would be remembered much after we are gone from this world. People would love us, respect us, and would be proud to be associated with us. It is extremely important therefore, to learn values from the parents and teachers in the childhood and follow good people of the society to make our life worth living, by doing good deeds like helping the society.

Learn courtesy, manners, etiquette, personal hygiene, dressing sense to add Elegance to your Personality.

It is understood that the type of a child's schooling, housing, nourishment, and overall upbringing is different, in every part of their world.

Nourishment of a child in a rich country, where an average parent can afford better things for their children, may not be same in poor or developing countries where average parents may be poor and cannot afford proper nourishment / schooling / food / shelter for the children or for themselves.

Out of Approx. 8 billion people of the world, at present, about 700 million people are extremely poor. These poor parents struggle to provide food and shelter to children and schooling. Proper upbringing and comfortable living, as is done in the rich countries, is a dream for these poor parents.

But the world is a very tough place, whether we have 'A Rich Dad or Poor Dad', we have to survive on our own when we grow up. And to survive well in this world, we have to learn the international standard of etiquette, courtesy, hygiene, dressing, and language to stay relevant in this global society and in any organization that we may be working in.

No one is bothered where we come from, what was our upbringing, which school or college we studied in. They want to see us as a good, well educated, well behaved, well dressed, well brought up, international citizen who can exist in an international organization, having modern lifestyle with emotionally balanced mind, a mature personality who respects all culture, language, religions, and all people of the world. In short, he/she should be educated, well behaved and elegant.

At a senior level, personal behaviour and professional excellence are most important

We work hard to climb the ladder. There are lot of hurdles, competitions, mysterious corporate factors and elements of luck, involved as we reach the senior position and eventually become the CEO, the Chief Executive Officer, of an organization. Two aspects, at this stage become very important.

- Professional competence and Vast experience
- Personal behaviour

Professional Competence and Vast Experience

At the senior level, one is expected to be highly qualified, highly experienced, and very competent to perform well as per the responsibilities. He/she has to take the organization forward, make the organization one of the best in the market in-terms of its financial health, reputation, and market share. His/her professional reputation and standing in the corporate world must be very high to enable him/her to maintain his/her position.

Personal Behaviour

The personal behaviour of an individual is extremely important at Senior Level, as you represent the organization as a senior executive. Besides, many people, including ladies and gentlemen report to you as your subordinates. You are a great authority and mentor for them. The entire organization watches you, your competence, as well as your behaviour which make you a great leader of the organization. The behaviour of a Senior person, in any organisation, is extremely important for a conducive working atmosphere, confidence, and loyalty of the employees.

In social life your good behaviour maintains your respect and dignity

Man is a social animal, we live in a civilized society, and there are neighbours, known and unknown people around us. We attend social gatherings, celebrations, various functions, meetings, etc.

We, therefore, meet people regularly in various areas on different occasions.

We must be decent, well behaved, well/properly dressed, as well as should be able to communicate well.

People feel comfortable with well-behaved and decent people. Polished behaviour therefore earns respect. Good communication skills, sense of good dressing up / attire, good etiquette and mannerism, makes a person, a respectable member of the society. The above-mentioned good qualities add elegance to the personality of a person. People are generally comfortable with such people.

Everyone wants well-behaved friend, colleague, neighbours, co-passengers, and co-workers as one feels comfortable with such people.

A well-behaved person is therefore respected in the society as an elegant and dignified person.

Behaviour, especially, with opposite sex must be always very good, decent, and proper. It is always good to maintain a safe distance, especially at the work place to avoid any kind of misunderstanding which might eventually affect the performance and also the reputation in the work place and also the career.

As a boss, one can be polite, respectful yet firm to get the task completed on time. Rude behaviour is repulsive and avoidable especially in modern era when we work with smart, enlightened, qualified and skilled employees.

Personal behaviour in a senior position is extremely important since this position is very powerful. One deals with lot of people, takes important decisions, lot of people report to him for their annual assessment.

Since the position enjoys power and is a decision-making authority, his personal integrity, ethics, language, maturity, and behaviour are extremely important. The way he/she deals with his/her colleagues, subordinates, the way he/she behaves, his/her emotional balance, his/her gestures, and body languages must be such that employees feel comfortable, safe, and happy to work with him/her.

Sober habits, gentle behaviour, mature and empathetic behaviour normally are well appreciated by the people.

A Senior Leader, therefore, has to be liked, respected and accepted by the employees as a highly skilled expert, a mature and trust worthy person as well as a great leader.

CHAPTER VII

How to Manage Relationships?

The most talked about topic and the most complex matter in our life, at present, is understanding and monitoring relationships. But alas, the truth is, those who are not in any relationship are in a hurry to get into a relationship, those who are already in a relationship have kept their 'fingers crossed' to maintain their relationships and those who want to quit it are in a hurry to get out of it.

We should know what is a relationship and why it is so important for human beings. Human beings have emotions, feeling of love, likes, and dislikes. Relationships are common in all living bodies, like human beings, animals, birds, insects. Even plants have relationships with insects. But human beings are most intelligent and understand the value of Relationships, better. We are also blessed to enjoy relationships for a longer period, provided we are mature enough to understand the value of it.

Relationships which are acquired by birth are permanent in nature and easy to maintain. Relationships with parents and other siblings are automatically good because they are blood relations.

Relationship with friends must be based on mutual respect. Similar habits and similar nature can promote a long lasting relationship. But most important relationship to understand, is the relationship which is based on attraction, love, trust, and commitment.

Relationship with opposite sex is a beautiful yet complex subject. Young generation, involved in relationship is prone to get involved whole heartedly. They may neglect studies, career, and even parents / families for their relationships.

An unsuccessful love related relationship can totally break a person, leading him/her to deep mental depression. Many have committed suicide because of broken relationships.

a) Relationship with parents.

Our first relationship starts with our parents, as we are connected to them since our birth. A baby establishes his/her relationship with mother, even when he/she is her womb.

The baby grows inside the mother, is nurtured by her inside mother's body. Once born, the baby becomes mother's most precious possession, who loves the baby, takes utmost care of the baby's well-being. The baby also receives lot of love from the father.

A child, therefore, establishes a great relationship with the parents. This relationship stays throughout life as both the parents and children love each other a lot. This relationship is based on mutual love and not based on any materialistic outcome.

Parents remain concerned about the children even when they are grown-up. Parents love their children more than even their own life. Children also reciprocate in the same way, as they also love their parents and know that the parents are their friends forever.

b) Relationship with the Spouse/ Partner

Relationship with the Spouse/Partner, with whom we spend our entire life, is a very important relationship of our life. Especially the spouse, i.e., wife or husband, is our life partner.

She / he sacrifices a lot to make her/his spouse happy. A wife leaves her own house, parents, siblings, friends, and comes with the husband to spend the entire life (as prevalent in Indian Sub-Continent). It is a Sacred relationship, which must be respected, protected with a lot of love and care. This relationship depends on mutual respect, adjustments, and trust.

After our parents, and our spouse are our closest relation. We have children and we establish our own family with our spouse. There are examples where a couple, husband and wife, have spent 60 to 70 years of long married relationship, with each other.

The present generation, however, is different. The economic independence of both husband and wife, lack of adjustments, tolerance, trust, and materialistic approach towards life have unfortunately, for some people, replaced mutual love, care, and feeling for each other causing Separation and Divorce.

Relationship with the Spouse/ Partner depends on mutual love and trust and is very valuable relationship. This relationship, if maintained well, provides a lot of happiness to people.

c) Relationship with Friends

People with similar habits become friends instantly. Slowly the mutual respect, and trust add to the higher level of relationship. There are friends for life, you can trust them, confide in them, and take their valued advice when needed. It is always a great pleasure meeting friends as you can share a lot of things with them and as meeting friends are always enjoyable experience. Real friends, though rare nowadays, will stand by you when needed, relationship with friends however depends on mutual understanding, mutual love, and respect as well as reciprocal support.

c) Relationship with the Organizations

As we start working in an organization, as employees, we automatically become a part of the organization. A relationship develops with the organization, which can last for a long time. A person can join an organization / industry as a Technician or Management Trainee at the age of 21-22 and can serve up to 60 to 65 years.

A person may join to serve in the Army (E.g. India) at an age of 20 and may serve up to the age of 60 years, as a Commissioned Officer. This kind of long relationship would depend on:

- Liking the organization and its culture
- Steady personal growth within the organization
- Loyalty to the organization
- Conducive working atmosphere within the organization
- Fair dealings by the organization
- Passion for a particular profession/Career. E.g. Some families in India, have been serving in the Armed Forces, especially in the Indian Army, for Generations because of their Passion and Patriotic mindset.

Romantic Relationship & Vanishing Treasure of Love

If there is any relationship which is sweet enough, long enough, and enjoyable enough after relationship we have with our parents, it is romantic relationship with opposite sex.

When a boy falls in love with a girl or when a girl falls in love with a boy, it is a romantic relationship because this relationship is based on romance, the love for each other.

For the first time, you realize that you like someone, who is equally confused, eager to meet you, and gives you tremendous joy and happiness whenever he/she is with you.

What is Romance?

It is feeling of excitement and mystery associated with love. Quite often, it is said that romance is a relationship between two people who are in love with each other but not married to each other. This may sound as if romance finishes once the couple is married. This kind of thought process needs to change. If one loves his/her spouse, the romance can continue throughout the life. There must be true love between the married couple based on mutual respect, sharing, caring, sacrifice, and trust.

A bit of fun, good sense of humour, a peck on the cheek, holding hands of the spouse, appreciating her/his dressing sense, behaviour, warmth, even mere presence in the house, singing few lines of his/her choice, reciting a favourite poetry, getting a gift to surprise her/him, sitting together for few moments, expressing love for each other, can be great moments of romance. Yes, romance must exist even between married couples, who are even married for a long time and must not vanish after marriage or few years after marriage. But for that, both partners must love each other, give proper importance, and care for each other.

We must love what we have and enjoy every moment. Love, romance, and happiness are our personal choice. Far away fields always look greener because we see the near ones always and can notice the negative points, ignoring the positive ones. But we have not seen the far away fields closely, hence do not know it's negative points. Let us learn to love what we have. Let us appreciate positive points of the person we love, ignoring negative points, as all of us would have some positive and some negative qualities.

Romance is a feeling of love. Holding the hands of the lover or spouse and is also being romantic, as expressing your love does not take much time. During pandemic, Work From Home, gave us an opportunity to understand the real value of our family and spouse. It provided the opportunity to bring back romance in our life, especially for middle aged and elderly people who have almost forgotten the meaning of romance.

Vanishing Treasure of love.

The romantic relationship has undergone a huge change. In today's world of materialism, advanced technology, economic independence and as everyone working in their respective profession, love has become materialistic, calculative, and success oriented. That innocent, emotional, crazy love for each other has vanished, when one used to travel miles to get a glimpse of her/ him, which gave tremendous satisfaction. When all effort to hold her/his hand, hiding from the inquisitive eyes of friends in a garden gave the feeling of walking in the paradise. When a hug was never so easy, when a kiss was very rare, and one was ready to sacrifice anything for her love. When lovers fought even with parents to get married to his/her lover. When love was more of a sacrifice, when love just happened, the entire world was non-existent in front of beautiful & most desirable girl/boy in the whole planet and one would do anything to get her/his company. When one would spend sleepless nights thinking about her/him, her/his beautiful face, hands, smile, fragrance, and touch (if one was lucky enough). Love was without any expectation, even at times, with doubtful result.

This kind of true love is fast vanishing now. People nowadays use more of head than heart while falling in love. They consider money, status, physical and materialistic happiness before considering love. The great treasure of true love is fast vanishing from the human life and with the arrival of the Artificial Intelligence, the experience of love may be synthetic without the element of crazy emotion, which used to make the feeling of love so pure, genuine, and divine.

What is Love

Love is an emotional and strong attraction towards someone, filled with sense of affection, care and likes.

The person we may love, could be parents, our spouse, friends, a special person, and also our pets.

In fact, love generates love. We love our parents because we know that they love us. We love some friends because we know those particular friends also love us. We love a particular person because we know that, this person, treats us differently, the language & gestures are different, eagerly waits to meet or talk, likes to spend time, feels very comfortable, and is genuinely concerned, has an unconditional feeling and caring for us.

We know how a pet, say a dog, loves us, his gestures from a distance, his special type of barking, his effort to jump on lap or to lick us, are his way to convey his feeling towards us, his love towards us. And he is extremely sincere, loyal as well as possessive.

Love fulfils a person's life. Love may happen before marriage or after marriage as one starts loving his wife or husband, he/she is married to. Love gives tremendous mental satisfaction. It automatically increases the sense of responsibility as one wants to do various things for the lover, who may be a friend, a fiancé, wife or husband.

The essence of love is that, one wants to make the other person happy. One is ready to sacrifice, anything to make the lover happy.

Earlier, people used to get married to an unknown person, and love or feeling for each other started after the marriage and couples, unknown before marriage, spent 50 to 60 years of married life together, as was prevalent in Indian sub-continent and may be with the fortunate ones elsewhere in the world.

The quality of adjustments, tolerance, and sacrifice kept these married couples together in spite of all kinds of problems regarding finance, health issues, more children, size of the family, different background, different culture, different type of upbringing. Love, thus, is the most precious possession of a person and only the lucky one gets the real, pure love, provided he/she knows how to reciprocate love and appreciate as well as respect the love and the lover.

The love, expressed in love letters, was a great source of expressing one's feeling and keeping the couples together though at times, they remained separated, stayed far away from each other due to job / business related issues.

Love Letters

Love is a Sacred Passion, is a Divine Gesture, a Ready to Sacrifice Attitude for the person you love.

Earlier, Love used to be expressed through Letters, to hide the Feelings from others, the inquisitive parties.

A love letter, which used to reach after a long and secret route, was read more than 100 times and kept close to the heart, kept safer than a bank locker.

The simple words of the love letters used to increase the heart beats and used to make one crazy and impatient to meet the lover.

The lovers took high risk to meet at a pre-decided lonely place and at times faced a lot of humiliation from jealous and wicked passers-by or even parents who invariably, did not accept or encourage their love. The lovers, quite often, exchanged love letters, as such meetings were invariably, short, to avoid inquisitive eyes and parent's scolding. The love, was a pure relationship between two lovers. The feelings, were kept secret at heart which was full of mutual admiration, likes and attraction. The love was without any benefit, unconditional and crazy.

Modern Relationships:

1.Marriage. Marriage is one of the best institutions. Based on mutual love, trust and sacrifice, the institution of marriage has lasted for generations. Many married couples enjoyed happy married life for 50/60 years and beyond.

2.The Concept of Divorce came with less tolerance, economic independence, lack of adjustments, etc., which was rare earlier.

3.Live-in Relationship. Live- in relationship is a new trend and depends on mutual understanding. It is a relationship, which gives a lot of pain when the relationship is broken. This relationship is not as strong as marriage and if not successful, it leads to a lot of mental depression. One should be very careful before deciding about Live-in relationship, because, in this relationship, both partners move in with mutual love but one of them may move out easily, if he/she, so desires, causing a lot of pain to the other partner.

Pandemic offered opportunity for love and prolonged honeymoon at home.

In spite of all problems, the pandemic directly or indirectly offered opportunities for extended honeymoon or renewed honeymoon for the married couple or couples staying together.

No morning rush hour as spouse or children did not have to rush to office or school or colleges. All were working from home including children attending classes On Line, which enabled the members of the house an easier morning schedule.

People did not need to dress up and get ready as they would otherwise do, during normal office, school or college days.

Very few people needed to dress up in formals, and a lot of time was saved as no makeup or formal dressing was required by the people as they were working from home.

Extra time for Romance During Work From Home (WFH)

One may or may not agree, but a little extra time, in between busy WFH, could be made available for additional romance, especially for younger couples, which under normal circumstance would never be available.

Singing a nice romantic song to the spouse who was working in the kitchen, could be real fun and an unforgettable experience.

Having a surprise cup of tea/coffee offered by the spouse just when we were very busy in a webinar or online conference was such a welcome and pleasant surprise.

All these small things between husband and wife, or couples, made the relationship more enjoyable, entertaining and stronger, during pandemic.

In our day-to-day normal life, the romance of couples or married couples was restricted to few hours after the day's work or on holidays.

The lockdown period, due to pandemic, offered all of us extra time for hobbies, as well as for romance.

As the couples stayed together throughout the day as well as night, and as outings, shopping, and all events including parties, get- togethers, were absent, the couples had all the time to themselves to rejuvenate their romance, a lovely experience, fast fading in midst of rude practical life, chasing the success in career and dream of more wealth, name as well as fame.

People miss the golden period of romance of young days in their advanced age as advanced or old age come with lot of more responsibilities, unknown physical and medical problems.

I am not suggesting to do romance by ignoring or avoiding office responsibilities, that would be inappropriate and avoidable. Good employees and executives work even more when not supervised, because they are honest and sincere. Organizations depend on them and trust them. However, Pandemic/Work From Home, did offer rare opportunities to couples, to renew their romance, since they stayed close to each other the entire day and it was a welcome change, though, during an unpleasant time like Pandemic.

Romance between couples can be done by saying few good things, appreciating each other, sharing lighter moments, few jokes, few enjoyable past experiences, helping each other during a 10 to 15 minutes coffee break or during a 30 minutes lunch break.

A shammer or a dishonest employee or worker is not liked even by the spouse or partner, because a dishonest partner will be dishonest even in any relationship, hence time spent for romance during office hours must be short and without compromising with office responsibilities.

Work From Home, at times, extends even after stipulated office hours, if international business partners are involved, because of change of timing across the world and employees work accordingly, without any complaints.

Quite often, Work From Home in MNCs involves longer working hours, and engagements even on a national holiday as MNC may be working in few other countries at the same time.

A short break for romance with the spouse or partner, therefore, can be a welcome break, to be enjoyed with a mature mindset and good sense of responsibility.

Effect of the pandemic in the domestic front affecting relationship

The pandemic forced locked down in all most all countries. All business activities including Industries, offices, malls, multiplexes travelling, hotels and restaurants schools/colleges everything stopped functioning. People got locked down at home. They somehow managed to purchase some household items to run the family, to provide basic food to family members.

During locked down period, the children were most affected as their schools and colleges were closed and they could not go out to play or meet friends.

Most of them hated online classes as they missed the fun of school/colleges.

The old parents also got bored as they missed their morning and evening walk and mutual friends in the parks.

Quite a few families faced tough time to run the family as the bread earners lost the jobs and families were facing economic crunch. Quite a few blue collard employees lost their jobs and many including white collard employees had a salary cut. The domestic atmosphere in many houses remained grim and unhappy. People were scared about the disease, bored staying at home and unhappy being jobless or getting less salary.

The relationship among the family members at times became strained due to the following reasons:

1. Family members lost jobs and families faced financial hardships
2. As all family members stayed at the house whole day, almost locked inside, people, at times, became irritated because of frustration, helplessness, unemployment, lack of privacy, etc (especially in a small house/flat).
3. Tolerating each other for a long time and elder's interference in personal behaviour,
4. Caused a lot of problems for the younger generation, as most of them wanted to be in a room, locked up with their laptop and mobile, as per the modern trends, needing more privacy.

Advantage of being together and increasing love, due to the Pandemic

The silver lining of the dark and unhappy period of Pandemic, however, was the opportunity of staying together, the entire day, during locked down period.

Ladies who were not working were used to staying at home the entire day, working in the house. They waited for the husbands to come back in the evening. Even the children came back in the evening from the schools/colleges. The ladies who were house makers/housewives, thus, at times, got bored and felt lonely the entire day. The pandemic however made it possible for all members including spouses to stay at home.

The lady of the house not only got the desired company but also helping hands in domestic chores.

Though the children started attending schools/colleges through online sessions and spouse or both husbands and wife were working from home and remained busy on desktops/pc/laptops/iPad and smart phones, the entire family was at home. The sheer presence brought lot of cheers to the family.

It was particularly a happy affair for families where earning members did not lose jobs or did not have a major salary cut.

As people stayed indoors, a salary cut of 25% to 40% could be managed by the family as everyone understood the plight of the economy. Salary cut was always welcome than losing the jobs.

So, as all the family members stayed at home, it was a wonderful experience for husband and wife as very few couples of the world would have enjoyed such prolonged togetherness, day after day, month after month in normal working condition.

The prolonged close proximity of husband and wife for the couples having good relationship was a welcome change.

Though for few, it turned out to be nightmare, as these unfortunate ones could not tolerate each other, for reasons, best known to themselves but for happy couples, this was a God sent opportunity to spend some quality time together.

Yes, people were busy in their work and we all realized that all of us were working for more number of hours working from home as the meetings could be held even in the late evenings, on Saturdays and even on Sundays if needed.

Virtual offices were working on 24x7 concepts.

But still in between the meetings, in between work, one could find some time to have a cup of coffee with the spouse, spend a few happy moments, help the spouse in whatever she/he was doing. Sing a song for her, standing on the kitchen door if she was working in the kitchen, crack a small joke for him if he was fixing a painting on the wall, etc. The bonding between husband and wife, got a real opportunity to get even closer which does not happen when we attend our office regularly. During normal office routine, we get ready by 8:00-8.30 am and leave for office, we hardly talk to our spouse properly, once in office, we get very busy in our office work, business, and with our office staff/colleagues, meetings. Quite often, we travel from office itself for our official appointments/business meetings. We all get used to it, at times even neglecting our family life.

The work-life balance is something, easier said than done. People who work 9 am to 6 pm cannot afford to take any liberty. They will have to give their 100% for their office work. The journey from home to office and back, depending on the city and traffic always remains a big-time consuming concern.

There are lot of people in this world who are unemployed, some of them are qualified and experienced yet do not get the job they would like to get. There are few who are fortunate though to get good jobs easily.

So, we all work on a tight rope on our day to day official work and must give our best to keep the job in hand otherwise we all know that there are plenty of people, waiting to replace us.

One has to be very careful therefore to even think of maintaining a proper work life balance.

It is not impossible but in most of the cases, it is extremely difficult.

Work From Home (WFH) and its effect on Relationship

The pandemic, due to covid-19, had forced people for the lockdown hence most had the opportunity to work from home. It is because of this reason the work life balance concept can now be tried by most of us, provided, we understand the concept of 'work from home' and work sincerely and honestly so that the organization we are working for, can get the similar result, compared to our physical presence in the office.

We can enjoy the domestic bliss, the close proximity of the near and dear ones, including the dearest spouse and the children, provided we work properly , from home , without observation by the Boss.

Work from home can only be successful if everyone works sincerely, with integrity. The joy and pleasure of being at home, enjoying the company of dear ones, can last longer if our performance of office work is proper and good, as expected.

However, Work From Home, imposed during pandemic, offered an ideal opportunity to married couples, throughout the world to come closer, cemented lot of unsteady relationships, enhanced sense of romance in many hearts, which were normally taken for granted. It offered many opportunities to the married couples of all age groups to enjoy marital bliss in a new manner, which for some, especially elderly couples, had almost vanished from their normal life, since running the family, looking after old parents were more important, given more priority, neglecting own married life. Married life for people over 50 years, more so for couples married for more than 20/25 years become routine, monotonous, boring, full of responsibilities, and less enjoyable. As a husband once remarked on a lighter note "when we were newly married, my wife used to smile at me, used to give kisses but now after 20 years she only gives instructions."

But we all know what a house wife, a mother goes through the entire day as She is on a 24 hour duty schedule, looking after the husband, children, old parents and the house. And unfortunately, a stage comes in life, when a good husband only listens to wife's instructions, in the house.

The life and lifestyle for people who are super rich or rich are different but for normal people, the massive responsibilities of children's education, buying and managing a house/flat, the thought of retirement, payment of EMIs of house, car, etc., keep the middle-class and the poor people, quite unhappy. The job and efforts to retain the job, keep people busy attending the office/business and maintaining the family. People behave like robots. Their personal life, especially the elder people, is almost without any love, romance, or even leisure.

WFH, had offered some quality time to these unfortunate elders, loaded with endless responsibilities, to enjoy the company of their spouse and children, while performing for the organization.

Though the pandemic has brought a lot of misery to the people of the world, the WFH concept, adopted by the various organizations due to pandemic, turned out to be 'blessing in disguise' for many.

Important Aspects of Work From Home Concept

The employers, organizations, and human resources departments throughout the world are facing a lot of problems as the young generation's workforce want flexible time, more time for enjoyment, work from home, and better pay & perks.

They are qualified, talented hence demanding. Retention of talents has become quite difficult in various organizations.

The work culture of the organizations and long working hours, the frequent travelling due work-related issues are creating serious problems in the domestic fronts, creating lot of misunderstanding, even divorce among married couples.

Keeping an ideal work life balance has become biggest buzzword in the work place.

Lady workers, especially, young mothers find it very difficult to meet both the domestic needs and organizational needs. Many of them leave their job, though deserving higher position in the professional life. The concept of WFH, being tried for last few years in the western world and tried and tested in many countries during the Covid-19 pandemic can help us in a great way.

WFH, concept must be understood properly by everyone, to make it an acceptable employment option. It must be understood by the employer, the employee, and the organization.

Employer's perspective

An organization is run by men, machines, money and technology. In fact, men manage all other ingredients of the organization. And if men have to work from home, then it is a cause of great concern for the employer. Firstly because it is a new concept, not normal, not enough time tested and secondly controlling employees at home, monitoring their work at home with family responsibilities, expecting the same work outcome or result, altogether, creates lot of doubt about the sincerity of the employee, about the work done, the target to be achieved, and the trust as well as the commitment of the employee.

Employee's perspective

The experience of Covid-19 shows that the employees were committed and the result of work from home was good. An average employee was happier and worked well. He/she was sincere and in fact, in most of the cases, worked harder, better, to avoid any criticism for lack of effort.

Employees could spare little more time for domestic needs.

Their presence at home meant a lot to the family.

They could save a lot of time, due to avoidance of to & fro journey to office especially in trains and busses, where it takes a long time. They could save the time of driving, could save petrol/diesel. Could have home food and the pleasant company of spouse, children, parents and domestic confront.

Most of the employees were very strict about the office work and the result and also with the office timing.

WFH, was a welcome break from a normal office routine.

A concept, which could be easily tried provided a few things in WFH, are followed for long term future expectance:

1. The spouse must learn to respect the official commitment of the working spouse. His/her respect in the work place must not be compromised by the behaviour/conduct of the non-working spouse. The working member cannot be and must not be involved in a domestic work during officc hours.
2. The children must be trained or controlled by the non-working spouse or parents of the working person, not to disturb him/her during office hours.
3. No neighbour should also be allowed to disturb him/her during office hour.

A few cases of Moon Lighting, that is working for some other organization, to gain few extra bucks, have been noticed by some organizations in past. This must be avoided as it amounts to 'Breach of Trust'. The employees may have to pay penalty for this kind of misconduct and some employees may lose their job as well.

Organization's Perspective

Some organizations permit work from home 2/3 days a week, some however may allow all the days a week.

A periodical monitoring of the aspect of WFH by the functional heads and the employer may be able to determine the feasibility of the WFH for a longer period.

Be it as it may, all of us, the employer, the employees, and the organizations need proper training, mature mindset, and mutual trust to make WFH, an acceptable norm in the organization.

We all must understand that we will only survive if the organization survives, hence WFH concept has to be or must be followed as if it is my/our own company or organization and I/we will have to ensure proper working of Work From Home, which must be profitable for the organization, in addition to the benefit the employees enjoy from WFH concept.

It must be a win-win situation for the employers, employees, and the organizations.

Renewed family bonding, the biggest contribution of the pandemic

It may not sound well enough to digest easily but yet the pandemic had also contributed in a very significant way in some areas.

One of them was is the enhanced family bonding due to the pandemic and its effect of lockdown, people were compelled to stay at home. They were either working from home or doing something of their own.

The entire family was staying together the entire day.

The working fathers were not going to office, working mothers were also at home, children had no schools or college.

The entire family was together from morning till night

It was, on the flip side, as if everyone was on a prolonged holiday.

A pleasant and happy domestic scenario, never experienced before.

Though people got bored at home, missed their outings, office, schools, colleges and friends, they woke up to the idea that the pandemic was a long drown affair and all family members were required to spend time together and tolerate each other for a longer duration since they were all at home. The lockdown period kept on increasing and also the fear of Covid-19 in the minds of the people.

People realized this fact that if they stayed at home, they were safe and staying at home meant all to stay and live together.

All of them, therefore, learned to share the work of the family as no servants/drivers/helpers were allowed.

People learnt new skills to keep themselves engaged like, cooking, music, reading (a habit fading fast), drawing and sharing the TV with others with flexible control of the TV remote.

Though the supply of groceries, fresh vegetables, and fruits were restricted, people started enjoying restricted menu but company of each other. Parents love their children and children love their parents, the living together the whole day had its advantages and disadvantages, especially with grown-up children but the family was together by the grace of pandemic.

The contribution of the pandemic in creation of domestic harmony is enormous.

It helped the love in the family to grow, the people again realized the importance of the family is a different way.

All of them stopped all family members from going out, all of them were concerned about each other.

They cooked together, ate together, played together, stayed together. It was almost like a long picnic at home enabling a very happy family bonding with full mutual love, caring and sharing, as well as mutual concern.

They noticed and kept on hearing from the TV/Radio how people were dying in millions around the world.

There was lack of medical facilities, hospital beds, even doctor and nurses, and worse a proper medical treatment ensuring safety from Covid-19.

Much talked about double shots also could not stop infection in some cases.

The family members realized each other's importance in the family and loved to stay together, united, and at home letting go a little bitterness, if any, of past. Each of them understood the value of life and clung to each other more closely than ever due to the scary new Corona virus variant.

Pandemic, though created great loss to human beings, economy and the peace of the world, inadvertently contributed to the great family bonding as the people were compelled to be locked down at their own home.

Pandemic compelled the family members to have breakfast, lunch, and dinner together, see TV shows together and spend more time with each other which had almost stopped in modern era, before pandemic.

Nowadays each family members remains locked in his/her own room. She/he is busy with the mobile, PC, or TV in his/her room, when present at home.

Most of us are busy from 9 am to 9 pm with our studies, business activities, career, etc., and stay away from the home leaving our parents and spouse at home for most of the day. Even on Sundays and holidays grown up children have their own agenda, own activities, mostly with their friends and stay away from parents.

Quite often, working couples also spent lot of time outside the house, being busy for their career, business meetings, office activities including official travelling.

In fact this type of official travel increases with the seniority and more responsibility in the organization.

This temporary separation, however, creates, avoidable distance between the family members especially with spouse, who might not be working or is compelled to stay at home because of old parents, small children or temporary illness.

Quite often a lot of misunderstanding develop due to the temporary and short separation. People also tend to become more independent in nature, and become less caring for each other or even develop could not care less attitude, which is extremely harmful for any relationship especially for married couples.

Being compelled to stay at home due to pandemic, yes it was understood that, vessels kept nearby, thus would produce some noise, but it was a 'blessing in disguise' as it has brought the family members, especially married couples nearer than ever before, i.e., staying in close proximity of each other. The husbands and wives may argue or even fight on some trivial matter but the inner love would bring them together eventually.

This enforced togetherness is the rare gift of pandemic which we must appreciate.

Working from home has become a new norm and it has lots of advantages like saving time on traveling to the office, spending maximum time at home with family, can easily look after old parents, can help the spouse in looking after the small children as well as household chores, apart from spending quality time with the family.

We should use our Brain as well as Mind for taking decisions Regarding Relationships and Career without being Emotional.

Some young ones of the young generations, at times, get infatuated or over-excited, and adopt some measures which are harmful to herself/himself.

In today's materialistic world a person should be smart enough and mature enough to protect herself/himself by using brain along with mind so that she/he takes necessary steps, against something which may harm her/him eventually.

Relationship at a young age is, unfortunately, very uncertain in present day scenario. A child falling in love at the age of 16/17 studying in high school is not sure whether he/she would be in some other country for further studies, as it is planned by parents. He/she may stay abroad for a long time, finishing the studies, and working for some time. The prolong separation, out of sight out of mind concept, all play a very important role in our life. Both the girl and the boy, while growing up, struggling to establish themselves, go through a lot of hardship and changed circumstances. The childhood love may or may not remain active. One should therefore, be very careful about taking some critical decision in early stage of life so that they don't repent in future.

And such critical decisions about own life cannot be taken by heart alone, one must use the brain also to evaluate and analyse the issue before taking a plunge.

Because at that young age of 17/18, parents take decision for the better career of the child as they love their child the most. They want to see their child well established in life and be happy in life.

Parents, all over the world, therefore plan the progress of their children.

Children, though, think they are big enough, hence must be extremely careful about their own safety, security and dignity, because in most of the cases even parents are unaware about the thoughts of their children.

Children, who take decision from their heart may at times, land in facing mental depression, unhappiness, tension which at times may lead to suicides, as young minds cannot tackle serious personal problems.

Young ones should therefore use both Brain and Heart before taking any long-term decision regarding their Relationships and Career, as we have only one life and it cannot be wasted by our improper decisions taken, based on emotion.

Important Tips for Better Relationships

No one in this world, can say for sure that he understands and knows everything about relationships, but few important tips, given as follows, may help the young generation:

1. Never be in a hurry for any relationship. Temporary likes and attractions to someone is infatuation. It is not enough for a mature relationship. Many relationships broke, even marriages broke for such hurriedly taken wrong decisions, which gave enormous pain to a person.

These kind of broken relationships make a person, lose trust in love and relationship.

2. Wait for the right age to get into any relationship. When we are in school or even in college, we are too young, impulsive and immature, we do not know the world. Our young mind may fall in love, can get attracted to someone but we must not forget our responsibilities, our studies, our career, our future, our dream and that of our parents who are waiting to see us become successful in life and look after them when they grow old. Relationship of love, needs commitments, which we can only fulfil when we have become successful in life, when we are in a position to take vital decisions, capable of looking after the loved ones.

3. Never compromise in a relationship because it will keep you unhappy, throughout your life. If you do not like something, say it now, let the other person know it. If your partner does not like something in you let the person say it, rather than keeping in heart and suffering for the entire life. One should be accepted as he/she is.

4. Be sure before your commitment. You cannot sacrifice everything for the happiness of one person, who do not even know for long. Loving someone does not mean, you ignore your parents and your family. Before you commit to someone think of your inherent commitment to your family, who looked after you so far and made you, what you are today, sacrificing their own comfort.

5. Once in a relationship, allow time for it to grow, do not commit anything immediately. First try to know each other properly. Think do you really love him/her, can you adjust with him/her, throughout your life.

6. The best way to take the love related relationship forward is to have acceptance from both the families. Your parents have sacrificed a lot for you. They will love

you forever, more than anyone in this world. Allow them, their say, in your life. You may be able to convince them, which will be the best solution.

7. Once in a relationship, respect the relationship, which is based on trust, love, respect and commitment. The partner must have enough confidence on you, on your love, on your commitment.

8. Love your partner with your heart and brain when you have decided about your relationship.

9. Give more power of opinion to your partner in your love life. Let the partner feel empowered, trusted and be overall authority of your life. No, I am not saying you become a slave, you must keep your self-respect and dignity, but the person you really love, make him/her your better half, and love her/him whole heartedly, sacrificing your own comfort, that is the secret of maintaining good relationship.

10. In our life, we play multiple roles. We are son/daughter, we are brother/sister, husband/wife, father/mother, employee/boss in our official career. We have to learn to maintain all relationships giving them equal attention, commitment and time to keep the relationship, stronger and longer. We need to sacrifice a lot to maintain a relationship.

11. Being sincere, loving from heart, showing respect, sacrificing own comfort or and giving preference, making the partner feel empowered, liked, loved always, are the key ingredients of relationship.

The word relationship is extremely important in present era as young generation get into a relationship quite early in life, and many of them suffer badly from the result of unsuccessful relationships.

Relationship is the way people, organizations and countries behave with each other. It is important to learn about the relationships and maintain the relationships for longer time.

CHAPTER VIII

What is Resilience and How to Convert Failures into Success in our Life?

Resilience is the unique capacity of an individual to recover from the failure or temporary setback and achieve success.

Resilience is the rare quality to learn from failure quickly and convert failure into success.

There are lot of things which do not happen as per our plan, or we do not get the result as per our expectation or unforeseen situation like the Covid-19 incident, which shatters our dream, puts us into a lot of trouble, financial, mental, emotional, and legal problems, etc. But we must have the courage, composure, patience, grit, and determination to regain our strength, thoughts, and special skills to fight back and win over the situation.

Success does not come easily and one cannot be successful every time, but the spirit of fighting back, a strong willpower to bounce back, can change defeat into victory, failure into success.

Few Inspiring Examples:

One such example is a person I know. He had few small shops, tea stalls, etc. He decided to buy a mall and run it properly. So he sold all his small shops and bought a multi-storied mall in the suburban of Mumbai, in Feb/March 2019. He modified, repaired, and decorated the mall in a very nice way. Lot of good brands opened their shops in the mall as it was located in a good locality, where lot of customers were expected every day. The mall started working from May 2019, when children had their holidays. The mall had sports arena as well as a lavish food court. A 4 storied mall with ample car parking.

The mall was doing very good business but it had to be shut on 23rd March 2020 when everything was shut, in India, due to Covid-19.

The family was devastated, with heavy financial debt. This person was frustrated, unhappy, and his health condition deteriorated.

His wife suggested to open one/two food takeaway service from own home to neighbouring locality, to maintain the family.

During Covid, no maid or servants, cooks, or any helper was permitted, nor they were available.

The Tiffin Service, with food items, started by this person, was liked by local community, which was tasty and cheap, became huge success with in a few months. He started few more outlets in some other areas. Today he has about 12 Tiffin service outlets. He has his own small tempo trucks, 2/3 cooks few delivery boys, one Manager to manage his business. And his business has become very popular because of the good quality, timely service, and cheap rates.

There are many examples like this, who succeeded because of their resilience during the bad days, during the pandemic in 2020-2021.

Many people lost their jobs, many businesses had to close down, many building remained incomplete, many types of business suffered causing unemployment of many people throughout the world.

But many people, using their resilience through their grit, determination, tried to do something new, something which could still be started during the bad period of Covid-19 and yet profitable.

Lot of people, became Entrepreneurs overnight to save their families from the economic hardship faced during Covid-19.

Resilience taught many people to start New Business and Source of Income during The Pandemic

Pandemic compelled lot of people learn the knowledge of Computers and Internet. As a lot of people lost their jobs, people started new On-Line Businesses with the help of E-Commerce.

The e-commerce and online new business could offer a lot of innovative business which could be different than traditional business and yet could offer a lot of employment.

For example, Online gaming business was increasing in leaps and bounds, and online entertainment business on OTT platforms, etc., became popular, hence some new business activities, keeping in view online viewers, could be thought off which could be planned by people, senior citizens, mothers/house makers with small children, staying at home.

Few Examples of New Business and Source of Income, which could be started by the people at home:-

Stock Market

With little effort and expertise, investment in stock market could be very useful. Investment could be done with small amount, after doing proper research of various companies especially Blue-Chip companies on the TV. One could become an expert in a few years and earn lot of money. Investment in stock market could be good source of parallel income in every house. Mothers with small children, retired people, physically challenged people and people with interest in stock market could not only earn a lot but also could keep themselves engaged in a positive way.

All could learn by trial-and-error method and become expert in a few years.

This extra earning could provide a lot of incentive at a time when a lot of people were unemployed because of the pandemic. The scope was enormous and many could be engaged in this profession, adopting it as the additional income or even main source income.

The trading could be done on line, on own computer, or on phone through some stock brokers or some stock broking agencies.

A detail study of various companies on the TV for few months, to ascertain their track record would enable us to decide which stock to buy. Low investments initially would allow us to learn more about buying of profitable stocks/shares, which may offer good return.

The gradual success would encourage the buyers in a great way and this profession could be an additional source of income for those who were compelled to stay, at home due to say small children, retirement, physical conditions, medical reasons and exigencies like pandemic, when many people had lost their employment and were almost locked in their own houses due to fear of Corona virus.

The Pandemic made people think of new opportunities for income.

It was an ideal time for the start-ups and small business to start with as many people lost their jobs and were forced to find alternative source of income to maintain their families

As I have mentioned about the trading business by house makers, retired personnel, and physically challenged people and many other people who were compelled to stay at home, there were many other businesses which could be started on line staying at home. Few, following Online Businesses, could be easily started:-

Private Tuitions

Expert teachers of various subjects could take private tuitions to teach students online on their respective subjects. They needed to connect with the students through internet like Instagram, YouTube, own website, etc. For example, if a teacher was very good in Maths and Stats, he/she could teach Xth, XIth ,XIIth , AS level and A level online to many students. They had to follow CBSE ,ICSE (Indian Boards), , IB (International Baccalaureate) etc. syllabus, on a particular link and time. He/she could take few classes in a day, keeping in view the difference in time in various parts of the world.

Teaching online by Private Tutors could start in one's own country first as the time factor could easily be managed, once popular, he/she could teach students of other countries near by, following proper syllabus.

Fees could be kept low as the number of students would be large, which would also attract many students.

One could start online teaching/coaching organization with the help of few teachers, teaching different subjects. A business which would require.

- Qualified, experienced, and passionate teachers
- A proper time table keeping in view the various different time of the world
- Sound knowledge of the syllabus of reputed universities / boards.
- A good internet connection with website, link, Wi-Fi arrangements
- A good publicity in the social media.

Expertise in Data Science and Data Technology

The Data Technology / Data Science was becoming very important in modern era. Obtaining a degree/diploma in Data Technology could give a huge boost to one's employment. One could then work from home using his/her expertise of Data Technology for many companies, until the situation allowed us to attend the offices. Data Science / Data Technology had become very important along with Cloud Computing. There were plenty of job opportunities for experts of Data Technology and Cloud Computing who could either start their own venture or work for well established companies even staying at home.

Teaching Music and Musical Instruments

Teaching Music or Musical Instruments could be a very good occupation from home especially during pandemic.

Music, especially classical music, could be taught by qualified expert music teachers following a proper syllabus and ensuring proper/regular practice sessions.

This was particularly important as the students were getting bored at home. Music, those who are interested, would offer a platform to learn and enjoy music removing the boredom.

Of late, a lot of adults had also shown interest in learning music as they wanted to pursue music as a hobby. They wanted to utilize the time learning music and singing for their own entertainment and that of their family members and friends.

Music was very good form of art; it purifies our mind and can entertain self and others around us.

A lot of young children wanted to learn music. A good music teacher, therefore, had a vast market to use his/her talent and earn as well.

Periodical test and friendly competition, as well as online musical events could be very entertaining, encouraging and would enhance the confidence of the learners.

Teaching music online could therefore be a good earning option.

Teaching a particular Musical Instrument could also be easily done online e.g. Violin, Guitar, Tabla, and Mandolin could be taught with little effort, provided the students were eager to learn and love music. Playing the strings of guitar could change the atmosphere of the house in a very positive way bringing joy and happiness. Playing Violin could make the home atmosphere so soothing and peaceful. Music could also attract lot of friends, who are interested in it. Music, therefore, could remove boredom and could keep the young ones especially happy and suitably engaged.

Human Resourse Management (HRM) Consultancy Service

One could be an HRM consultant through online HRM consultancy service, provided he/she was properly qualified with sound knowledge and experience.

The apps like LinkedIn could help in getting data of people seeking jobs in addition to own contacts.

A list of people seeking employment could be made keeping in view their expertise, qualifications and area of interest.

One could use the corporate contacts to know about the vacancies existing in a particular company or any other HR requirements.

For example, online Tele-Interviews could be conducted to shortlist the eligible candidates and forwarded the company's HRM Head or the CEO for final interview.

A suitable commission could be earned accordingly.

It was a good option for working from home and starting own venture as an HRM consultancy. It was a nice way to employ yourself and help others to get employment. Once established, it could grow into a Permanent Organization.

People's Resilience and own initiatives during Pandemic

Pandemic offered tremendous opportunity for Start-Ups who could start a venture and operate from home using internets.

I have seen few ladies starting their own home-based restaurants and supplying regional food items, especially liked by a select crowd particularly their community and thus maintaining their families, especially selling to some single parents, who were looking after their children and parents, elderly couples, etc, during these difficult days, and who needed ready-made food.

Some of them were smart enough to understand the food habits of people staying nearby and made food items according to the choice of particular community or particular region who used to or like certain types of food.

For example – English menu / Continental menu, Mughlai menu, Chinese menu, Italian menu, Lebanese menu, Japanese menu, etc. and in a vast country like India, Punjabi menu, Gujrati menu, Bengali menu, etc.

Special & Regional menus provide enormous opportunities to the small home-based restaurant owners to supply cooked food of particular menu to the particular crowd and could easily run their family during the pandemic, when their spouses, fathers, themselves, the bread earners of the house, may have lost their jobs due to the lockdown.

These kinds of start-up trends could be possible in all major cities of the world. Some people, might be working/staying temporarily, some of them may be students but most important part was that all these people from various countries missed their home food and if someone could reach out to them offering them home food and delicious menu of their choice, the particular start up could easily survive.

Ethnic culture, language, and food habits were a common bond among people. It always increases friendships among people across the world, forgetting Borders of the Countries. It gives a great feeling.

I would like to share a small incident here.

We were on a Trip to England some time back and we were taken to Lake District of UK for a day's visit. We were taken to a restaurant for lunch where the owners were from Bangladesh.

We were a group of 32 people from India and traveling with a reputed travel agency.

As my wife and I were speaking in Bengali we were surrounded by few people, including the owner of the Restaurant. They asked us, if we were Bangladeshi and we told them that we were from Mumbai, India.

They again asked if we were Bengalis and we said yes. They owners were so happy that they not only spoke to us for 10 minutes but also ordered extra sweet dish for all 32 of us, free of cost.

We were shocked, taken aback, and embarrassed by this kind gesture of the owners. We knew we would not meet them again and were unable to return the favour, but the owners, who were from Bangladesh, did not listen to us. They said they were lucky enough to meet us, the Bengalis, and they were delighted to look after us.

The common language and common culture, thus, have tremendous emotional connection and can make the World Border Less.

The home-based Start-ups with regional menu and ethnic connection, therefore, had bright future especially during pandemic when people were locked in their homes and unable to visit the restaurants of their choice.

The power of Resilience developed New Generation of Entrepreneurs with new Start-Ups

A lot of graduating students were also thinking of new Start-ups. A good idea can enable us to start our own business, own entrepreneurship.

Since e-commerce was doing well during pandemic, a lot of online business in the fields of logistics, supply chain, restaurants business, entertainment business, gaming business could be started, provided you had some brilliant and innovative idea.

We could use internet to our great advantage and for the e-business.

As pandemic had led to the lockdown and we all were compelled to stay at home for own safety. E-business or online business offered abundant opportunity. There were plenty of things the world wanted, the customers and consumer wanted, there were a lot of services which could be provided by online business.

The entertainment business had tremendous opportunities to explore. Especially on OTT platform. If we all thought about the area of our expertise, we could come out with some online business ideas which could be started as Start-ups.

Few examples of instant Entrepreneurship during Pandemic.

Sometimes we behave desperately when we are put back to the wall.

Here are few examples of instant entrepreneurship :-

1. Ms Sonia (actual name changed) got her Offer letter for a good job, from a good company during Campus Placement Interview in mid-March, 2020. She was to join from 1st June 2020, after her final exam of Software Engineering

The national lockdown was announced on 23rd March 2020, in India, due to Covid-19 and the entire nation came to grinding halt.

By mid-June 2020, about 5,00,000 people died due to Covid-19 in various countries of the world. The advanced countries like USA, UK, Germany, France, etc., struggled to check the disease. The medical infrastructure even in these advanced countries were found to be insufficient.

Ms Sonia could not join the job, and the company decided to reduce man power due to lockdown. Ms. Sonia, was in huge problem. Her father's business, a small restaurant, in the suburb of Mumbai was shut due to lockdown.

The family of 4, i.e., Sonia's parents and a younger brother had to be maintained, a few outstanding payments were supposed to be made by her father, but could not be paid due to no income for few months. The Restaurant staff had to be paid their salary as a minimum strength of staff had to be kept for the restaurant, waiting to open in a few weeks.

Ms. Sonia, now a Software Engineer had excellent knowledge of Computer.

Ms. Sonia, decided to start her new Enterprise, a new online business to impart basic computer training, Online, to home makers, the ladies staying at home and who were not working outside, due to family commitments and small children, as well as old parents. Their husband were working outside but due to lockdown, most of the husbands had either lost their jobs or lost their business or were working from home

Ms. Sonia, named her company 'Elder's Computers' and gave her advertisement in Instagram, Twitter, Facebook, YouTube, etc., her USP was:

- Elder's Computers is an On-Line Classes to teach Basics of Computers.
- It is easy to learn basics of computers
- People of any age can learn
- To remain updated, all should learn computers
- Proficiency in English language was not required
- Course especially designed for ladies staying at home, to educate them the use of computers and internet.

- Duration 8 weeks
- Fees INR 10,000 can be paid in 2 to 4 instalments
- Timing 5.30 pm to 7.30 pm, Monday to Friday from 1stAugust, 2020. She gave the advertisement in social media in last week of June 2020 and was flooded with the request by mid-July for the course which was to start by on 1st August.

She started the first batch of 30 ladies on 1st August, 2020, where the ladies borrowed computer from their husbands, and children at a time (05.30 pm to 7.30pm), when computers could be spared easily. Seeing the increasing number of students, Ms. Sonia started the second batch from 2.30 pm to 4.30 pm for people who could manage to have a computer during that time. Only 30 students were allowed and rest were asked to join from 1st of October, 2020, 2.30 to 4.30 pm and 5.30 pm to 7.30 pm from 1st October, 2020.

Thus, she conducted two courses for 2 batches of elderly ladies and also elderly men, each day, Monday to Friday.

She did not need any money for her Start-up, used her own laptop and smartphone to teach the basics of computers and internet.

Money started coming in the family. More and more elderly ladies and elderly men, who were staying at home, thought of being upgraded and teach savvy, joined the course offered by Ms Sonia.

The word spread from mouth to mouth and Ms. Sonia became the talk of the town.

'Elder's Computer' became famous in a very short period. Pandemic, thus, offered few opportunities for the people who had ideas of new Start-ups.

Sing Friend Sing.

Aadil completed his International MBA in September, 2020. He tried to get a placement offer since June, 2020, by attending interviews in few reputed companies. Finally, he cracked an interview in October, 2020, for Assistant Sales Manager in a well-known shopping mall in Mumbai. He was to join by 15th Nov, 2020, as the situation due to Covid-19 was improving and malls, restaurants, etc., were reopening, since India had its festive season approaching. Companies normally did good business during these months in India, i.e., from October to December. In 2019, it was said that Amazon made a business of **3 trillion** USD during Diwali in India.

So Mr. Aadil was very happy, and joined the mall on 15th October. Slowly the business was returning to normal, and economy was looking up due to great demand even for luxury goods cars, TV etc.

Aadil, fresh from International MBA course, took, a lot of interest to learn the job and establish himself in the new setup.

He received lot of appreciation from his bosses because of his sincerity and customer care activities.

As things were going well, and he kind of settled in the company, he decided to marry his girlfriend in Dec 2020. Aadil's family included father a retired school teacher, mother, Aadil, and two younger sisters studying in junior and senior college.

Now married Aadil, could help his father to run the family as he was working.

In January 2021 the second wave of Covid-19 created havoc in UK and the second wave of Covid-19 started effecting India in a big way. In Aril 2021, the pandemic aggravated very strongly in India with more severe intensity of Covid-19.

Various parts of India faced lockdown many people were dying due to lack of oxygen, ventilators, hospital beds.

Business activities went out of gear, malls, restaurant, gyms, salons, multiplexes got shut, travelling reduced drastically.

Mr. Aadil lost his job as malls got shut. He had the responsibility of a big family including his newly married wife.

Aadil was totally shattered. He had to earn to run the family but how?

Once again everything stopped working the economic activities stopped and unemployment become a huge problem in the whole world including India.

Aadil could not sleep few nights, though his wife Alia kept on telling him that things would soon be normal and that he should not be depressed and lose all hope.

Aadil was restless. He kept on thinking for an alternative source of income.

One evening, since they were just married, Aadil and his wife Alia were spending some time together on their terrace and Alia requested Aadil to sing a song. Alia was constantly trying to keep Aadil busy in conversation of other topic rather than employment and bad days. She wanted to see him happy.

Aadil, had learnt Indian classical music during his school days and could sing well. He could also play a few musical instruments like harmonium, guitar, and piano, etc.

On being requested time and again by his newly wedded wife, Aadil sang a small 'Ghazal', a melodious song, based on one of the best Indian Classical 'Ragas' with lyrics written in Urdu. The lyrics were ---"Phir wohi shaam, wohi gham wohi tanhai hai, dil ko samjhaane teri yaad chali aayee hai."

The song, translated in English should be something like this

"Once again, the similar evening, similar sorrow, similar loneliness have surrounded me, and to pacify my heart, your memories have come back (which have made me even more sad). An excellent Ghazal Sung by Ghazal Maestro, Mr Talat Mahmood .

Alia started crying and told Aadil that he sang really well.

Aadil got up and took Alia to the dining room for dinner. Aadil could not sleep that night. All of a sudden, he got an idea to start a new business, a new Start-up, which could be done staying at home, on his laptop, with no investment.

Next morning he launched his new venture, an online venture of Teaching Music. He made a website and gave publicity of Facebook, Instagram, Twitter, You-tube about his Start-up. He named his Start-up as 'Sing Friend Sing', a project which included following:-.

- 'Sing Friend Sing; – would try to teach the music lovers few Ghazals, light Indian Hindi songs, and basics of musical instruments like harmonium (needed to sing Ghazals), Piano and Guitar etc, On Line.
- Age limit 16 to 60 years
- Duration of course 6 months
- It will only try to teach students the basics of music to enable them to gain confidence to sing and develop themselves to be better performer with own practice, at a later stage.
- The aim is to encourage the shy music lovers to sing for themselves and for their family members and friends
- To enable the students to utilize their free time in a positive and creative manner and promote own talent which is unused so far.

- To introduce students to a good hobby like singing and not only listening to music which everyone does.
- There will be two tests, after 3 months and 6 Months
- It is an online course, so personal laptop or computer (desktop) is required
- The fees was INR 18,000 INR 6,000 should be deposited as initial payment, on enrolment
- The enrolment would be done by Mr Aadil Mohammed, the MD of 'Sing Friend Sing' company.
- Students will benefit more if they have their own harmonium/piano, or guitar.
- The online classes will be from 10.30 am to 12.30 pm, from Monday to Friday
- The link will be provided to attend the session, after enrolment.
- Classes for first batch of 20 students would start from 1st July 2021 from 10.30 am to 12.30 pm the second batch also may start on the same day in evening hours from 5.30 pm to 7.30 pm, depending on demand of students.

Aadil started his publicity on 15th May, 2021 and by 30th May had 120 students were ready to join him, eager to learn music.

Most of the students were ladies of age group of 40 to 60 years.

The first batch started on 1st July, 2021, and became an instant hit as lot of people came to realize that singing was so self-entertaining and such a good pastime as well as hobby.

'Sing Friend Sing' became a great success story. A fantastic initiative taken by talented young man, Aadil, which could make a lot of people happily occupied in their creative and entertaining hobby, i.e., singing.

It was a hit among especially elderly people who love music like Bhajans (songs about praying to God) and Ghazals the melodious romantic songs, mostly written in Urdu and Hindi, and are extremely popular in Indian sub-continent and among the people of Indian sub-continent, settled in various parts of the world.

Both Bhajans (Religious Songs) and Ghazals were sung by with the help of 'old musical instrument', Harmonium or Piano as these instruments matched the natural tone, texture of human voice. People loved to sing Bhajans of Chanchal and Anup Jalota and others as well as Ghazals of Jagjit Singh and Pankaj Udhas (Great Indian Ghazal Singers) as well as Mehndi Hassan, Gulam Ali (Great Pakistani Ghazal Singers) to name a few.

These singers had been performing in front of packed stadium, whenever they performed in their own country or abroad.

'Sing Friend Sing' therefore became a massive hit as a unique start-up of Aadil.

Maths for all

Rahul Sawant, a brilliant student, had to go through a very difficult time.

After completing his Ph.D. in Maths, Rahul managed to get a Maths Teacher's job in a private school with IB curriculum in Mumbai in September 2019.

Rahul was very thorough in his subject, which was not a pet subject for many.

In India, students join college for 4 years graduation course after completing standard XII or 'A' level in IB curriculum.

Rahul found that most of the students were weak in Maths, and therefore, were very scared of the subject.

The standard of students was also different as they studied in different Boards, for example, State Board, CBSE, ICSE, IB, etc. Some of them lacked in basic knowledge in Maths, since quite a few did not like the subject.

Rahul, realizing this, wanted to help the students to gain the basic knowledge of Maths and also tried to bring all students to same level of standard so that teaching could be easier and assimilation could be better. But the colleges closed on 24th March. 2020 due to National lockdown in India because of the Covid-19, Pandemic.

As it was a private college and Rahul was still not confirmed, he lost his job as schools and colleges remained shut for uncertain period.

As economy of India as well as the world was bad, many people lost their jobs, many schools and college found it very difficult to survive as many students could not give their fees on time because their parents either lost their jobs and were surviving with slashed salaries.

Many organizations including schools and colleges tried to function with online sessions due to lock down and cutting cost wherever possible.

Rahul was also one of many such people who had lost the job, which he had just started enjoying.

He was the elder son of a family consisting of mother and two younger siblings, He had to find a job fast but as everything was closed he had to sit in his small apartment, thinking what to do. Rahul, while teaching found that generally quite a large member of student were weak in Mathematics and Statistics. Quite a few take additional tuitions from private tutors or coaching classes to even pass the exams.

Rahul thought of starting an online Maths coaching class for students from 8th standard to 12th standard including AS level and A level.

He named his venture 'Maths for all' trying to tell the students that no one should be scared of Maths as it needs average intelligence, which all students have. It needs dedication, determination and practice. All students following these simple principles can score good marks. He gave out advertisement in social media saying the following:

- 'Maths for all' is an Educational Start-Up, an On-Line Maths Classes, to enable even weak students understand Maths in an easy manner and score good marks.
- Once enrolled in the course, passing will be very easy for even the weakest students as it will be, if needed, one to one coaching to teach basics, remove doubts on one to one mode and solve many question papers to provide confidence to the students.
- There will be two batches in a day from Monday to Friday with 25 students each from 10.00 am to 12.00 pm and 4 pm to 6.00 pm
- Fees INR 3,000 per month, per student from 1st July 2020 to 30th April 2021
- Fresh batches will be enrolled from July 2021 to April 2022.
- Initially each student has to pay Rs. 9,000, i.e., two months tuition fees in advance in addition to the fees of July 2020, the fees paid in advance which will be adjusted for the month of March and April 2021.
- Enrolment will be done in portal given in website on 'first come first serve' basis, starting from 1st June 2020 for batches of 2020-2021

- The link to attend the class will be provided to the students before 1st July 2020.

Rahul's 'Maths for all' became a massive hit as 50 students for two batches were enrolled up by 10th June 2020. Request came to start the third batch on the same day which was declined as Rahul wanted to see the result of first two batches during the final exams. Rahul started his venture sitting at home, without any investment or infrastructure. He just needed his laptop and a white board to take the sessions.

The power of Resilience in our life therefore can elevate us from a bad situation to an extremely good situation. But we will have to make an endeavour to turn around our bad time into good time.

As Shree Vivekananda, the famous saint cum philosopher had said.

"Rise, awake and stop not till the dream is accomplished."

There are bad days and good days in our life, but we will have to survive for us, for our children, for our family.

In the Indian sub-continent and few countries in Europe, some countries faced problem of Partition of National borders, as a result millions of people were displaced. We saw trouble in West Asia where thousands lost their home, properties and became refugees overnight. Recently thousands were killed and many were displaced again due to trouble at Ukraine and Gaza.

So incidents like Spanish flue, Covid-19, World Wars, Geo-political troubles in addition to devastation due to floods, Earthquakes, Volcanic Eruptions, Tsunamis, etc., will happen time and again, disturbing the life of innocent people and their families. Only the power of resilience can save us and bring us back to the normal life.

Resilience Taught us to learn new skills, during Pandemic, for keeping us happy, indoors.

Pandemic had kept all of us at home. Even people who were working from home had extra time as they saved travelling time, time to dress up, particularly for the work place etc.

If planned well, we would have some time to learn or practice new skills, as mentioned below:-

Cooking

Cooking, a skill which many of us would love to learn. All of us eat and many of us were used to getting ready meals, courtesy, mother or sister or wife. Quite a few of us did not know proper cooking and worse, did not appreciate the effort and hard work that needed for cooking.

We had seen, in our childhood, our mothers cooking. A mother cooked with lots of love for her children, she cooked dishes which were liked by the children. Mother, at times, gave away the entire cooked food to children, even going without food. She loved to watch the children relishing the food made by her, which gave her the maximum satisfaction.

Cooking therefore is an act of love and affection. You cook for someone you love so why can't we also learn how to cook, because, only then, we can show our love to the people we love, including our parents, spouse, children, even friends.

Learning cooking may also enable us to offer a helping hand to the people in the house who were cooking usually. It would be a nice gesture to help the family members in cooking. A kitchen, we should know, is Not Gender Biased.

Cooking is therefore a nice skill to develop while staying at home for a longer period. It is an art if mastered, could get a lot of appreciation and accrue lot of self-satisfaction. Cooking for our loved ones, gives us an opportunity to show our love to the people, we really love.

Learning Music

A lot of people learn music at various stages of life. Some, who are very talented, learn music in their childhood, some learn at a later stage, as enough time to pursue this wonderful hobby called Music was not available earlier. One can learn classical vocal music, or can learn musical instruments like guitar, sitar, violin, flute, etc.

If one had learnt earlier or is now seriously interested, one can learn and practice. Music is self-entertaining and can keep us busy for hours in a very positive way with lots of self-entertainment and fun. Music is good for health and mental health. Music purifies our mind and keeps us happy. It is a nice stress buster. If we do humming or singing, whenever we are alone, we would feel mentally happy.

Learning Dancing

Like music, dancing is also self-entertaining. Classical dances are not only very beautiful, it is very satisfying for the performers.

Dancing keeps a person physically fit. Indian classical dancing like Bharat Natyam, Kathak, Manipuri, Kathakali, Kuchipudi, Odissi, etc., are difficult to learn, beautiful to watch and tough to perform. Ballet is yet another graceful dancing. Waltz with your partner is such a nice dance. Dances like Jazz, Hip Hop are also popular dances.

All forms of dances keep people physically fit, mentally happy. This hobby is also self-entertaining as well as Pandemic offered enough time to learn and practice dancing, a nice hobby and good physical activity.

Dancing is an excellent combination of graceful and beautiful expression and good body movements. A good talent and an entertaining hobby, which is appreciated by almost everyone. People who take to dancing remain physically fit forever. It is therefore a fine art, entertaining for others and healthy for the performer.

CHAPTER IX

Important Ingredients for Holistic Development.

Holistic Development of child is extremely important to be successful in life and to be capable of playing multiple roles in his Personal life as well as Professional Career.

To have a happy, healthy and successful life, the holistic development of a person is very essential.

Some of the important aspects, required, for Holistic Development are appended below:

Proper Education

Proper Education helps a person in proper and good upbringing, mature behaviour, liberal, and broad mindset.

Proper Education, make a person a civilised, disciplined, law abiding and ethical citizen, who is an asset to the society.

"Education is the most powerful weapon which you can use to change the world"—Nelson Mandela

Everyone should therefore be educated for own benefit and also to be a useful citizen of the world.

Sports and physical activities

In the era of advanced technology people from their childhood get used to laptops, desktops, cell phones, tablets, TVs etc.

They spend most of the time, in a day, using the above-mentioned gadgets.

Understood, that these gadgets are very essential tools, at present, to survive in our day-to-day life, but they have their negative aspects as follows:

- These gadgets make us lazy, chair/sofa bound
- Reduces our physical activities
- Deprives us/our young ones of Outdoor sports activities/outdoor physical activities, which are very important for our health, fitness, agility and entertainment.
- Make us a loner. We have started living alone in our room with these gadgets. Today father, mother, and two children sit in a room, busy with their cell phones, not talking to each other. The gadgets have made us a loner, friendless and self-centred, uncaring, unloving and anti-social.

We must, therefore, adopt some sports and physical activities like playing football, basketball, walking, jogging sports, etc., to keep ourselves physically fit or else very soon, more people, even young ones, will have deceases like Diabetes, Heart Problem, Blood Pressure etc. which will take place due to our sedentary life style.

Sports also teaches us various qualities like skills of team spirit, leadership, co-operation, collaboration, sacrifice, camaraderie etc. which have a lot of benefit throughout our lives.

Physical activities would make our life happier, healthier, disease free and even longer.

Creative and self-entertaining hobbies

Hobbies in our lives are like oasis in a desert. Hobbies give us much needed, self-entertainment, solace, a little space we need in our life and develop our talent and promote our creativity.

If we pull a few strings in a Guitar, after a day's hard work or sing a few songs in a quiet corner, play instruments like Sitar, flute or any other instrument of our choice, it gives us immense pleasure. A little time, spent in our hobbies, is very refreshing and enjoyable. Hobbies are very self-entertaining and since it gives us internal happiness, we feel like continuing for few hours. Music is a hobby which can very easily keep us engaged for few hours on a holiday or whenever we have a break from our work.

Painting sketches, sceneries, portraits can easily keep us engaged for a few weeks, if we have time.

Drawing an abstract painting of own imagination is so fulfilling, entertaining and creative as well as satisfying.

Composing music is extremely creative and entertaining. It stretches our talent to a different level.

Hobbies like gardening can also be so satisfying. You would love to speak to the plants when saplings grow big, you can feel the happiness of the plant, when it is looked after and nourished properly. The beautiful Rose, your latest possession, a new rose plant with beautiful flowers, can keep you engaged, looking at its beauty for long time. You may admire the size, shape, and the colour of the Dalia for a long time.

Hobbies are our personal friends, they give us so much happiness. All of us must have some hobby, especially in this world of technology where real happiness is fast disappearing giving way to artificial happiness through technological gadgets.

Hobbies are our lifelong friends. Hobbies helps us especially in our old age, when we are alone and not very many people want to talk to us.

Indulge in social service

Helping the society, the people of our society is our responsibility and not charity. The society gives us a lot, only very few of us understand it, realize it and are thankful about it.

Warren Buffett, one of the richest men, in the world, has already given a lot and announced to give all his wealth for the welfare and help to the society and its people. He has said that he made this enormous amount of wealth from the people of the society and he owns his success to the society hence decided to give it back to the society.

We all must also remember the kind assistance we have received from the society and its people, we must also help the needy, the sick, the poor and the helpless people of the society with whatever we can like money, in kind, with assistance, as a mark of our gratitude to the society.

As we grow up and become successful in our life, we must feel that it is our responsibility to help the society like great people like Warren Buffett, Bill Gates, Mother Teresa, Florence Nightingale and many others have done. Let us do something for the society and it's needy people and keep our foot prints for next generation to follow.

Managing Work-Life Balance

Life at present has become very busy and very demanding. People leave home early and return very late, the professional life is very demanding. The work place, in most of the cases, follows 'No Mistake' syndrome. As a result people are extra careful, work harder to keep their jobs intact.

The number of unemployed people is very high in every country especially in developing countries and over populated countries. People, who are employed, are constantly, worried about their EMI's for car, house, children's education etc. They cannot afford to lose their jobs.

Another important point is the extremely busy work schedule and frequent travelling for work by senior professionals, it disturbs the domestic bliss.

It is worse if both husband and wife are working. Industries and business are global now. The life of working professionals has become very busy but they are kept happy with good salary.

But more time spent in office or office related work, causes unhappiness of home.

The Work From Home (WFH) concept has not been adopted by many organizations in all countries. The recent phenomenon of 'Moon Lighting' has become another avoidable practice by many employees which also cautioned the employers against work from home concept.

The present generation is used to a lot of luxury, entertainment, enjoyment as most of the parents are earning well. This generation, as employees, want more freedom, flexible timing in office, more leisure period, more entertainment and more time with loved ones, near and dear ones.

The work life balance has now become biggest buzzword in an organization. Since it is extremely important to keep and maintain a happy work force, the organizations are worried to improve the work life balance, to minimize attrition or losing good talents.

It is therefore very important for all of us to prioritize our needs with utmost maturity, giving equal importance to the family as well as the organization, we work in, so that we can maintain a win-win situation balancing our working hours and family life.

How to remain healthy in our life

The average lifespan is increasing because of improvement in medical treatment, quality and development of improved medicine and better as well as modern medical infrastructure.

All of us want to live longer, with good health.

Remaining healthy, however, depends on us. Our daily routine, our life style, our habits and our food habits are important to ensure our good health. Following measures may be helpful:

1. Early rise and early sleep. Early risers are more active throughout the day hence remain healthy. If we sleep early, we can get up early, more easily.

2. Daily physical exercise for at least on hour is a must to keep our body machine properly functional. During morning hours or evening hours, we must either go for a walk or jog for 40 min and do some free hand exercise / yoga for 20/25 minutes to remain fit.

3. Controlling the diet, we must be careful about our diet. Fatty / oily food, red meat, more carbohydrate should be avoided.

4. Avoid if possible or control consumption of alcohol.

5. Avoid smoking at all cost ,reduce, if you cannot stop totally. You can stop it. It is your strong will power which is required to stop smoking. Please compare the

pleasure of smoking cigarettes to the benefit of living longer (The benefit, would involve your career, family and happiness) and decide.

6. Avoid few things totally
   - Drugs
   - Unprotected sex, especially with strangers
   - Excessive drinking on special occasion (you may not see another occasion), so please do not do it.
   - Over enthusiastic dancing on a dance floor / pub, etc., when not warmed up (especially after 40 years of age). It is very important to note, please dance gently for 20/30 minutes and get warmed up for more energetic dancing, if you wish to do so. Please do not try to copy young ones, your advanced age and physical condition, may not permit that.

7. Get medical check-up done every 6 months, especially if you are beyond 40 years of age. Consult your doctor for the tests to be done.

8. Avoid heavy food at dinner.

9. Have your dinner before 7/8 p.m. daily.

10. A post dinner walk of 20/30 minutes, is advisable

11. Try to sleep well at night. Following steps for good sleeps may be followed:

   a) Do not go to bed thinking about any critical/complex matter
   b) Avoid any argument with your spouse or any one before going to bed
   c) Do not over eat before going to bed
   d) Keep your laptop, Cell phone at a safe distance
   e) Use comfortable clothing for sleeping

f) The bed, particularly the pillows, should be proper to enable you to sleep well

g) The night lamp should be hidden and kept at the proper place, only to help you, if you have to get up at night to go to washroom.

h) Adjust the room temperature of AC for your comfort accordingly.

i) While going to bed, try to forget unpleasant things of today and do not think about tomorrow.

j) Think about any good thing that happened today or in last 2/3 days and feel happy to have good sleep.

k) Don't drink more water just before going to bed or else you may have to getup sacrificing your good sleep and you may have to struggle to sleep again, thereafter.

l) Before going to bed, think about 5 minutes regarding things to be done as a routine like switching off lights, locking the door, switching off the TVs etc., so that you do not have to get up again, spoiling your sleep.

12) Last and most important thing to remain healthy, is to have a calm and peaceful mind. Follow ethics, be good and helpful to people, do not cheat anyone, be sincere, respectful, and do good to the society. Don't be jealous, avoid hatred and learn to forget and forgive, you will remain healthy and happy.

Follow Rules, Regulations and laws in our personal and professional life.

We stay in a civilized society, we stay among other people, we work with others in organizations. We can only stay safe, secured and happy, if we follow the social norm "Live and let live."

Every individual in the society has the right to live well. Everyone enjoys similar privileges in the society. Everyone also has the responsibilities to ensure that the society functions well to ensure safety, security and well-being of all members of the society.

Every country, therefore, follows the various laws, rules, regulations, required to ensure that all citizens are comfortable, safe, secured and are treated equally well.

The Govt, state administration, police and judiciary based on the guide lines given in the Constitution, work to ensure well-being of the citizen.

It is our duty, therefore, to follow all rules, regulations and laws of the country so that all our fellow countrymen are happy, safe and comfortable.

E.g. if we jump a traffic signal, while driving a car we may cause an accident and may cause discomfort to others in addition to own discomfort and penalty.

Following the traffic rules therefore is important. Similarly in case of personal life, domestic life and professional life we must follow

- Ethics
- Laws
- Rules
- Regulations

To lead a peaceful and comfortable life

A shortcut may result into a long drown legal procedure and penalty which may spoil our peace of mind.

It is very important that children from their young age are taught to follow all laws, rule and regulations in their personal, domestic and professional life to maintain comfortable, peaceful life and respectable life.

No room for Mediocrity

'Winner takes it all'. In life, we must try to be the winner, be successful. Mediocrity will never help us. We must excel in the field of our choice.

"We are what we repeatedly do, excellence then is not an act, but a habit." -Aristotle

We must therefore be habituated to excel and that will automatically catapult our performance to a much higher level and make us successful. Mediocrity, therefore, must be avoided.

Respect Others Culture, Language and Religion.

We are all global citizen now, we may belong to one country, study in some other country and work in some other country, anywhere in the world.

We will be working with many colleagues, who would be from other countries, would speak other languages and follow different religions and religious beliefs.

We will have to learn to co-exist with other colleagues, understand them, respect their culture, religion, and language, and form a homogeneous team, to produce better results.

Our individual likes and dislikes, habits, must be improved to accommodate and enable us to adjust with others, to survive in this global environment.

Be a good citizen of your Country and the World

The advanced technology has made the world, a small village.

We can communicate with anyone, in any country, we can reach anywhere very fast. The industries and businesses are all global.

Being part of global working team, we must represent our country well, hence we must become a good citizen of our country in respect of behaviour, etiquette, manners, education, so that our colleagues abroad, appreciate us and feel comfortable working with us.

At the same time we must also follow international norms, learn to behave as international citizen by learning various aspects to become a good international citizen. We must make our country proud with our behaviour, performance and good deeds, when located abroad.

Be a balanced, matured and unbiased person

If we follow discipline, if we work hard, we will be successful in our life. We may become Senior Executives, Chief Executive Officers, Chairman, and even great leaders.

And at that senior level, we will be in authority to decide about the fate of many subordinates.

We must be balanced, matured and unbiased to treat our colleagues, subordinates, and all employees well.

Every business is global now, we will be dealing with many people across the globe, being balanced, matured and unbiased, would make us more acceptable and respectable team member or even a great leader.

Be empathetic

Empathy is understanding other's difficulties and imagining ourselves in other's place and feel how others are feeling.

The world, at present, has approx. 8 billion people, out of which 700 million people are very poor. There are a lot of people who are not happy because of lack of money, their sickness, unemployment, and many others issues. We need to be considerate towards other people and our colleagues, our work force. An empathetic person can make an unhappy person happy and can make an organization a great organization with his maturity and great quality of handling the workforce.

Elevate your next generation to a higher level

It is our responsibility to elevate our next generation to a higher level. We have heard about 'Rich Dad and Poor Dad'. We may be born in a poor family, in a not so developed environment, but we must keep in mind always that with our passion, dedication, and hard work we can change the fate of our family and the next generation. If we become successful in life, with our hard work, we can change the lifestyle of our future generations and elevate them to better living, better lifestyle. Everyone must realize that it is of no use blaming our parents and predecessors, but with our own effort and hard work we can offer all the comforts to our present and future generations and elevate our next generation to a higher level. E.g. A car driver works hard and makes his son an Engineer or a Doctor. His hard work and sacrifice has elevated his next generation. It is our responsibility, therefore, to elevate our next generation to a greater and higher level.

Case Study No 2—Lift the next generation to a higher level (A true story)

Ms Santhia Gangadharan was born in a middle class family, staying at Chandrakant Niwas, Dharavi, in Mumbai. Father Mr S.P.Gangadharan, had his own business, was working hard to maintain a family 4 members. Mother was a housewife. Santhia had an elder brother who was studying Engineering.

The cost of food for 4 members, the payment of electricity bill, Water bill, cooking gas bill and cost of education of the children etc was a huge burden on Gangadharan. Santhia was good in studies. She completed her Graduation (BMS) from a nearby college with good marks. Gangadharan and his wife wanted their children to study and stand on their own feet properly.

Santhia saw her father struggle to maintain the family, she also saw how difficult it was for her parents to bring up 2 children. She wanted to see her parents happy always. She decided to work hard, study well and become successful some day and with her brother, relieve her father of his huge burden. She was ready to sacrifice her comfort to change the status of the family by achieving something spectacular in life.

As she graduated with good marks, she wanted to study Masters in Management Studies (MMS), which is known as MBA elsewhere. She got admission in MMS(Finance), in a new college known as Guru Nanak Vidyak Society's Institute of Management(GNVS-IOM), near her house, at Sion East, Mumbai.

GNVS-IOM, was only 2 year old Institute when Santhia took admission, but it was good in quality of education, with highly qualified and experienced faculty members and excellent Chairman Sardar, Mr. Manjit Singh Bhatti, as well as Trusty Members. I was also fortunately involved in starting the

Institute as a Founder Member and served as The Chief Adviser and Faculty Member.

Santhia worked very hard and at the end of 2 years she secured The Second Position in MMS (Finance) Exam, in University of Mumbai in 2014.

It was the day of great achievements for GNVS-IOM also, which secured First, Second and Third Positions in MMS Exam of 2014, in University of Mumbai. A rare achievement for an Institute of Management which was only 4 years old. Ms Sneha Subhash Sanjiskar secured First Position in MMS (Finance), Ms. Santhia Gangadharan secured Second Position in MMS (Finance), and Mr. Mohammad Fahad Khan secured Third Position in MMS (Operations). Ms Shivani Sharma also of GNVS-IOM, secured First Position in MMS(Finance) in 2015 in University of Mumbai.

Santhia made her family, teachers and the college, GNVS-IOM, very proud, because of her spectacular achievement. The family became very happy due to Santhia's hard work and determination to uplift the family to a more respectable status.

Santhia thus enhanced the family's prestige and lifted the next generation to a greater height of aspiration, as the future generation would try to follow her example and climb greater heights.

Q1. What prompted Santhia to work hard ?

Q 2. How did the family benefit due to Santhia's success ?

Q3. How was Santhia's success useful for the next generation?

Ans of Q1.

Santhia loved her parents a lot. She felt sad and helpless seeing her parents , trying very hard to offer comfort to the children and the family.She always wanted to see her parents happy. Her father really worked very hard to maintain the family of 4.

She wanted to achieve something great to make the parents and the family happy.

She therefore decided to work very hard and become successful in life with her dedicated and determined effort, even at times sacrificing her own comfort and make the family proud of her.

Ans of Q2.

Since Santhia, a girl from Dharavi, Mumbai, secured the Second Highest Position in the University of Mumbai, in MMS Exam in 2014, the family came to lime light. People came to meet Santhia with flowers Bouquets, Gifts etc. The family became famous overnight. The family, all of a sudden, gained importance among friends and relatives.

Santhia, her father, Mr. Gangadharan, her mother, and her brother, everyone in the family became very happy as Santhia was honoured and appreciated by her College, GNVS-IOM, and University of Mumbai. Infact she along with other Toppers were congratulated personally by the Hon'ble Vice-

Chancellor of the University of Mumbai. The prestige as well as the status of the family increased. The Gangadharan family became happy and proud because of Santhia's hard work and ambition to succeed.

Ans to Q3.

Santhia's efforts were very important to set an example and become an inspiration for the future generation. She also realised that maintaining a family of 4 members kept her father on the toes always. Santhia saw her father working very hard. The expenditure for clothing, requirement of more food, more rooms to stay since Santhia and her elder brother were growing and needed more privacy, the cost of education in higher classes/ colleges, were too much and her father was the only bread earner at that time since her elder brother was also studying.

Santhia wanted to reduce the tension, to some extent, by securing good result in MMS. A great thought of a growing child. Santhia wanted to work hard and become successful in life and set an example for the next generation to also work hard and achieve success which would ultimately enhance family's prestige and elevate the family's status.

Santhia took a lot of interest from the begining of the MMS Course. She was very regular in the class and followed the teaching and directions of the professors, very sincerely. She kept her focus on the studies and was determined to do well.

She thus secured Second Position in MMS Final Exam, in University of Mumbai in 2014 and Created History, for a girl from Dharavi, known to be an underdeveloped area of Mumbai, having inadequate facilities.

Santhia;s tremendous hard work, dedication and determination to make the family proud and lifting it to a more respectable level, was Very Praise Worthy. Santhia;s hard work would also inspire the next generation to work hard and achieve success in life like Santhia did. The end result was good for the entire family and it's future generation.

CHAPTER X

What is our Life's Goal/Aim?

The famous Hindu Religious Books, Upanishads, speak about 4 Purushartha, goals of human life.

1. Dharma (Righteousness)

Dharma is righteousness. To be honest and do right things.

An example of following Dharma.

Emperor Ashoka, in India, conquered Kalinga State after a fierce battle, where a lot of people died and got injured. Wherever Ashoka used to go, he used to see people crying, as most of the families lost their male members in the battle. He became very sad.

He became almost a Saint, opted Buddhism, following the Great Religious Leader, Lord Gautam Buddha.

He sent his own children to other countries to spread Buddhism, wishing no one would fight a battle in future, so that people are not killed and families are not destroyed.

Emperor Ashoka followed Dharma because his Heart and Soul told him that he had no right to kill so many people, even though he was the Emperor.

Countless people died because of him, since he wanted to conquer the kingdom of Kalinga, to establish his supremacy, as the Emperor. He realized that because of him, lakhs of families got destroyed and devastated. Lakhs of females became widows; the children lost their fathers.

Ashoka realized his mistake. He therefore adopted the path of Dharma, the path of righteousness, and decided to shed violence forever.

2. Artha (Prosperity, Economic Values)

3. Karma (Pleasure, Love, Psychological Values)

4. Moksha (Liberation, Spiritual Values, Self-Actualisation)

People in ancient time followed these principles and tried to achieve these 4 goals of human life, at least in Indian sub-continent, one of the oldest civilizations of the world.

The goals of our lives in modern era, are quite similar to what Upanishads, conveyed. These may be as follows:

- Education
- Financial Stability
- Career
- Family
- Self-Development
- Social Responsibility

Education

As we all know, education and educational qualifications, make us better human being. Education is now the measure of good citizen and also a yardstick for a good career.

An educated person like a doctor, engineer, professor, etc., enjoys a good career and respectable life.

Financial Stability

Financial stability enables a person good standing in the society. Financial stability uplifts the living standard of a person and makes his family members comfortable in life. The family members can afford better things in life, get better quality of education, enjoy luxurious items to use and are considered well established in the society.

Career

Everyone has a career in the society. Some have a better career, with better economic condition, prestigious designation, better positions. Some people do not enjoy that good career and struggle to get established in a good career. But one of the life's goal of all of us, is to have a career and we all work hard to have a good career. A good career elevates our prestige in the society, makes us financially well established as well as makes our family happier.

Family

One of our main goals is to look after our family, i.e., parents, spouse and children. We must ensure that our family members are happy and comfortable. That the young ones receive good education so that they have a good career when they grow up. We must make sure that family members have good and enough food, education, medical benefits / medical insurance coverage, and all necessary items/things, which are required for comfortable living. It is our duty and responsibility to elevate our family to a higher status, by our hard work, so that next generation can be proud of us.

Self-Development

Self-Development is a continuous process in this fast-changing world. Parents have provided us with basic education. But it is our duty to learn new skills, acquire new qualification to remain relevant and to take our career to a higher platform.

Social Responsibility

We must understand what society has done for us or does for us continuously. Society's contribution is enormous for all of us. It is therefore, our responsibility to look after the society, by giving back to the society. We must contribute to look after the needy, sick, and poor people of the society. We should try and make few unhappy people happy by helping needy people with money and our service as Florence Nightingale and Mother Teresa have done and Mr. Warren Buffet and Mr. Bill Gates are doing. Giving back to society is not charity but it is our responsibility.

What is the Aim of life?

As we plan to have a good, successful and meaningful life, we may follow few suggested guide lines:

- We must prepare ourselves well to become a good person, good son/ daughter, good husband/ wife, good Father/ Mother, and good citizen of the country as well as the world.

- Parents prepare us initially with basic teaching, learning, guidance, etc., but as we grow up we have to learn to prepare ourselves following the good examples of the society so that we become a good member of the society.

- Do our duties as a member of our family and also as a member of an organization we work in. As we grow and become big and mature enough, we must do our duties for our parents. Parents in old age need our help, we may be present in our country, or outside our country, we must help our parents and be with them when they need us. The same goes for the organization we work for; our duties and responsibilities must be fulfilled properly. The interest and the requirement of the organization is most important and we must ensure that we are useful to the organization and we help the organization to grow. Our sincerity, dedication and loyalty to the organization must not be compromised, ever.

- A very important aim of all of us is to fulfil our responsibilities to the society as well the country. The society contributes a lot to our life; hence it is our responsibility to contribute to the society's welfare and help it's people.

- "Ask not what your country has done for you think what you can do for the country", said John F. Kennedy, Former US President. We must do our bit to help our country through discoveries, research and service, etc., so that our country becomes stronger, richer and more powerful, as well as its people, become comfortable.

- To be a spiritual person to help the people of the world. We should try to become spiritual person, rising beyond our religion, as a spiritual person treats everyone of this world in a similar manner. We should become global citizen and help the people of the world irrespective of the caste, creed, culture, religion, even country like Mr. Warren Buffett and Bill Gates of US are doing.

- Do good deeds and leave our footprints for the next generations to follow. We should learn to do something very good, something spectacular, so that people can remember us for a long time even after we are gone. Like Albert Einstein, William Shakespeare, Abraham Lincoln, Mahatma Gandhi, Nelson Mandela, Rabindranath Tagore, Leonard Da Vinci, Beethoven,

Mozart, Isaac Newton, etc., who have helped the world and people benefitted from their work.

- To fulfil our responsibilities as per our various roles, we play in the world
  1. As a son or daughter
  2. As a brother or sister
  3. As a father or mother
  4. As an employee
  5. As an employer
  6. As the boss of the organization
  7. As a member of the society
  8. As a citizen of the country
  9. As a citizen of the world

We should work hard and up-skill ourselves to be successful, happy in life, and respectable in the society.

CHAPTER XI

What your life wants from you ?

Follow Ethics

Our life would be smooth, happier, and hassle free if we follow ethics in all walks of life, may it be personal, domestic, or professional.

E.g. If we jump a queue in a theatre in a mall, people would object, we may be picked by a cop and waste more time and face harassment. A shortcut becomes, invariably, a long cut.

If we don't follow ethics in our business, sooner or later the auditors, Enforcement Directorate, Regulatory Bodies would catch up and impose more penalties. There will be more loss of money and reputation. While trying to save a few bucks, we would pay more or even may lose license for being unethical. Being ethical would enable us to be happy in the long run.

Work hard to be Successful

We enjoy our success more if we have worked hard to achieve it. The journey towards success is remembered for a long time, the difficulties, the uncertainties, more and more hard work for ensuring success is cherished for a long time. Hence, fruits of success achieved after hard work is more enjoyable.

Try to perform well always, in a 'No mistake' syndrome

The world accepts only successful players, there is a 'No Mistake Syndrome' everywhere. Your performance therefore, must be excellent in which ever field you may be working in. You have to excel.

As former president of India, Dr. Abdul Kalam, has said, "Excellence has to be routine and not an accident". We are in the world where "winner takes it all" hence, we must perform well to be winner.

If you help people, God will help you

We are taking about Life Management Skills, in this book. There are lot of people in this world who are poor, badly sick, physically disabled, mentally retarded, and even orphan who are without parents or any near and dear ones. These people cannot manage their lives. Quite a few of them, in fact about 700 million people out of about 8 billion people of the world at present, are extremely poor. They are without food, clothing, and even shelter.

We, as human beings, have some responsibilities towards them. Hence, while learning the management skills to manage our lives, to become successful, we should also remember that there are lot of people who cannot manage their lives, they need our help.

We must help these needy, sick, and helpless people to make their life a little better. We should help such people with money or in kinds, to make them a little happy and if we do so, the God almighty would shower his blessings on us, which would make us happier and even more successful. Let us not lose the opportunity to help a poor man, a needy or sick man as his 'thank you' would bring us a lot more happiness.

We must also help the needy people of the society as it is our responsibility, as the society and this wonderful earth, the God's wonderful creation, gives us so much. Hence helping poor and needy and sick people of the society is our responsibility and not a charity. This act of ours will make God happy, and he always helps and blesses those people who help poor, needy, and sick people.

Be Properly Qualified, Skilled and be Competent.

We have to acquire proper qualifications and apt skills to be qualified, competent, and efficient for our tasks and responsibilities to perform well, always. The organization and its people are depending on us, the employees, for success and progress. The Performance Quotient (PQ) is extremely important in business world as well as in the industries. Our performance will only take us to the top of the ladder. Mr Satya Nadella, the CEO of Microsoft, and Mr Sundar Pichai, the CEO of Google, are the good examples for all of us.

Look after yourself with Healthy Practices

God has gifted us with this beautiful world and wonderful life.

It is our life and it is up to us to make our life a happy, healthy, and peaceful with our good and healthy habits so that we can enjoy this gift of God, our life, for a long time with good health and happiness.

Daily physical exercise, proper and healthy diet, a proper and positive mindset as well as enough sleep at night, are few important ingredients of healthy practices, that may keep us happy and healthy.

CHAPTER XII

How to remain Young for a Longer Period?

From our childhood, we work hard to be successful in our life. We study hard to get good grades in the school or college.

We work hard in our work places to climb the ladder of success.

As we grow, we get married, have own family of spouse and children. We again work hard to make our family happy and comfortable and at the same time be successful in our work place or in our business.

It is the irony of fate, that before we realize we grow from 20 to 30, 30 to 40, 40 to 50, 50 to 60, 60 to 70 years of age and so on. Though the difference between 20 to 30 is negligible, the difference between 30 to 40 may be felt a little more, but difference between 40 to 50 is a lot as we get into our middle age. The energy level and the agility starts reducing at this point.

As we grow from 50 to 60, we are unable to do lot of things which we could do in 30s & 40s. Age of 60 and above is considered advanced age and the society and its people start treating us differently. A lot of people Retire from their Work/Service, at the age of 60.

As we grow from 60 to 70, we are considered old. Our 70 years old body may have some problems. Lots of people have body ache, knee pain, eye problem, many may have blood pressure, diabetes, hypertension, etc., which may reduce our movement and normal activities.

If, by the grace of God, we reach 80 and beyond, we carry all the qualities of 70s, good or bad, including health issues. We are known as Super Senior Citizen and our movements become restricted in 80s. We must be very careful at this stage of life with our food habits, physical activities, etc., so that we do not become bed-ridden.

Quite a few old people stay alone, in their flats/houses as their children may be working out of stations or even abroad.

They have to be extremely careful in moving about from one place to another and preferably should have a helper along with them.

They should have a SMALL CARD KEPT IN A CHAIN ON THEIR NECK, in which their name, cell no., home address, and contact no. of spouse, son, daughter, or any neighbour, their blood group, name and contact number of the family doctor etc., should be written which may be very helpful in an emergency, especially when they are out of their house.

We have no control over our growth. We keep growing in age from our childhood to old age.

The physical changes in our body, the declining level of energy, agility, movement is a normal phenomenon.

It happens to all of us. From young age to slowly but steadily we reach advanced age and face the effects of advanced age.

We enjoy this stage of our life, the old age. We enjoy financial stability because of our life long earning and less liabilities.

We enjoy the respect shown to us by the people, being senior citizen or super senior citizen.

We also face the hardship of the old age. So how do we remain young for a longer period so that even when we are in 70s and 80s we remain young, we feel young, and can still enjoy in this wonderful world of God, to a great extent like a person, much younger in age enjoys.

How to remain young for a longer period?

Few Suggested Steps to Remain Young for a Long Time

There are few things, we must do to remain young for longer period:-

- We must do some physical exercise every day. Preferably, one hour in the morning. We may do a 40 minutes of brisk walk and then, do free hand exercise for 20 minutes. It will be great if we can do yoga for another 20 minutes. Yoga increases inner strength of a person, it makes nerves and inner organs of our body, work better. It enables Liver, Spleen, Kidneys, Heart, Eyes etc function better.

  This routine should continue, till we can walk. And if we follow this exercise regime from the age of 40, we will still be able to walk in 90s as our body will be used to this physical exercise regime.

  We must avoid walking on road, because of the traffic, or vehicles, the parks/fields are the best places to walk.

- Meditation is another good habit which helps us in many ways. It helps us receive cosmic rays and energises our body and soul. It increases the power of concentration, makes us mentally and spiritually strong as well as make us a better person. Meditation for at least 40/45 minutes, daily, can be really great.

- Follow an ethical life style. A person who is honest and follows ethics is a happy man without any worries. He is naturally lively, energetic & happy.
- No excessive smoking or drinking. Smoking is not only dangerous for our health, it reduces energy level in a person. Excessive smoking must be avoided to have a longer life and to remain young and energetic for long time.
- Excessive drinking is also dangerous for our health. It is very important to drink (if one likes to drink) within limit. We must learn to enjoy in our life and live longer with good health. Let us not permit our addiction enjoy us and make us imbalanced, less energetic as well as shorten our life.
- Adopt some hobby like singing or playing musical instrument. This kind of hobby keeps us young, energized, and happy. Our friends, relatives and anyone known to us, would appreciate our hobby. Hobbies make us adorable in the society.
- Play some games, we should continue to play some games with our children, even when they are grown up and we are old, with our grandchildren and our friends. Keeping in view our age and energy level, we can play, chess, cards, ludo, carrom, badminton, table tennis, etc. Playing games with own children and grandchildren would keep all family members happy including us, the old ones. Playing games like cards, chess, carrom, etc., with our friends of equal age would keep us happy, joyful, and busy in a positive way.

Playing games would not only keep us physically fit, but also mentally alert and happy, as we would spend some valuable time with our dear ones.

- Meeting friends every evening for playing some games is an ideal way of keeping ourselves busy. Interacting with dear friends, sharing past memories, sharing some mutually enjoyable jokes, would keep us young and happy.
- Be a helpful person. In the advanced age of our life, we must be helpful to all. As people respect us being an elderly person or being an old person, it is our duty to help the young generation, in whatever way it is possible.
- Do good deeds and remain happy. In our advanced age we should try to remain happy always. If we do few good deeds by helping, poor, needy, sick, or people who need any kind of help, we would remain energetic & mentally young.
- Pray to God whenever possible for his kindness and endless blessing for keeping us alive to be old enough, for enabling us to enjoy the long journey of the complex life and yet keeping us happy, and for his kindness for helping us throughout our life when we needed divine help in our most difficult days.
- The most important learning of life is to feel energetic, feel young, feel satisfied, feel happy for your achievements (and you only know your achievements and the difficulties you faced in life whether others acknowledge it or not), and be always ready to meet the God, the Almighty.
- Keep yourself engaged in a positive or creative activity. Old age, especially after 70, is a very lonesome age. People would hardly speak to you, they won't take you seriously. There may be avoidable criticism at home, even your so called 'achievements' in life may be devalued, you almost become a non-entity.

- It is, therefore, extremely important for the older generation to remain engaged in some positive, creative activity so that we can live peacefully and happily, spending some long hours in a day, doing something that we like to do.

I see one retired gentleman in our society, who engages himself in gardening in our large housing society, spread over 7½ acres of land, i.e., about 30,000 sq. mtr. of land. The housing society has multi stored buildings and stilt car parking as well as open car parking. But there are a few areas left for a little gardening and there are some fruit trees and trees full of seasonal flower, some extra areas for small plants. It is a nicely planned housing society with a huge lawn, playing areas for kids and gardens. This retired gentleman, a retired Army Colonel, takes very keen interest in sowing seeds, tree saplings, watering, etc. During rainy season, we see him with gloves in hand, cap on his head, wearing a raincoat working in the gardens of our society. He even spends own money to buy good plants from nearby nursery, so that residents can see some good flowers and enjoy neat and nice garden. I see him always smiling, happy and enthusiastic, a great example of social service and remaining young, energetic and happy.

- We see a lot of Hindi classical singers or Ghazhal singers performing in their 70s and beyond. The effect of music, the desire to perform well, the applause and appreciation of the audience, keep them fit and young. Bharat Ratna Pandit Ravishankar, the famous Sitar Player, gave his last performance at California at the age of 92. Recently, Ms. Asha Bhosle, the Famous Indian Singer, performed at Dubai on her 90th Birthday. Their superb talent, willpower to entertain people, their determination to perform well and tremendous love of

- the people, enable them to perform, remain young, youthful, energetic, gracious and gorgeous.
- I never agreed with the people who said our youth is short lived. I do not agree with the people who say they are old at 70s, as I feel that:
- "We may be of advanced age but we can still be young." We may retire but we are 'Not Waiting to Die'. We may still remain active and should contribute to the society.
- If we do good deeds and not harm or cheat anyone, if we pray to God every day and express our gratitude to him for his endless blessings and benign help, we will remain young even in 80s & 90s.

A clean mind, a clear head, a good hobby and a helpful attitude would keep us young for a long time.

How to get rid of Smoking and Excessive drinking to Lead a Healthy Life

We all know that smoking and drinking, i.e., smoking cigarettes and drinking hard liquor like Whiskey, Rum, etc., are injurious to our health.

Our lungs, oesophagus inside our throat, and our mouth are not meant to receive smoke generated by smoking tobacco. Such smoke containing Nicotine is bad for our body organs and blood.

There are warning signs on every cigarette packet that 'Smoking is Injurious to Health', still there are lot of people in this world who smoke ignoring the warnings, which are meant to warn them against smoking.

There are people who smoke 40 to 60 cigarettes a day. There are students in the colleges & universities who wait for a break every one hour to have a smoke, there are various professionals, and senior executive who smoke frequently, spending lot of money for costly cigarettes and harming their own health. The percentage of smokers are more in the countries where temperature during day and night is less.

Smoking, in real terms, does not provide any warmth. It is more of the psychological feeling that cigarettes are providing warmth. Some people feel comfortable while smoking in cold weather. In any case, smoking of cigarettes, lasts only few minutes and it cannot provide warmth for a long time. The little warmth lasts for a very short period even if one is 'chain smoking', i.e., smoking cigarettes more frequently.

I myself, a Retired Indian Army officer, served at a place on the Indian border, located at a height of about 16000 feet above sea level. The temperature at times reached minus 20 degree Celsius. I found non-smoking troops equally comfortable without smoking. In fact, they were more alert and were not restless or uncomfortable when cigarettes did not reach them, or due to heavy snowfall, when cigarettes were not available to them for a short period. Smoking habit was in any case, an avoidable habit in high altitude area, due to availability of less oxygen in the air.

Also, smokers, were less energetic as compared to non-smokers and at a high altitude of 16000ft height and beyond, where oxygen level was less, non-smoking made breathing more easy.

Even in our normal life, in normal areas, people who are involved in professional sports like marathon running, athletics, Basketball, Football, Boxing, etc., where high level of physical energy is required, smoking is avoidable as it reduces energy level of a person.

Smoking affects lungs, throat, mouth, and quite often becomes the cause of disease like Cancer, a dangerous and life-threatening disease.

People who do not smoke are better off as in present era, the smokers face a lot of problems at airports, in the hotels, malls, etc., because they have to go to an especially kept room to smoke, as most of the public areas are non-smoking zones.

Why do we start smoking?

One may start smoking for the following reasons:

- To know the taste of smoking
- To look smart and impress upon the friend/colleagues, especially the junior or young ones
- At times to avoid boredom/ loneliness
- To prove, in a friend circle, that one is growing up
- As a result of peer pressure, in a friends circle, where everyone smokes, 'I should also smoke or I will become a social outcast'
- It is a part of attraction in adolescence period of a child, when he wants to try out various things.
- We want to copy some film stars, who smoke in the films and look very smart and stylish. A lot of young people tried to smoke and follow a renowned Hindi Film actor known as , 'Pran', who used act and smoked in all most all his Hindi films and he made smoking quite attractive among young generation in 70s-80s with his unique smoking style. Some people also tried to follow famous Hollywood actors in Hollywood movies, showing their great style of smoking while acting.
- Once we start smoking, it becomes an addiction and we begin to smoke regularly.

How to Leave Smoking

We all know that smoking is an addiction. It is very difficult to leave smoking. People hide and smoke in the bathroom, when not permitted to smoke in open area, they hide cigarettes packets in the car to avoid scolding from parents and even spouse.

A lot of people smoke even in the old age as they tried to leave smoking but failed to do so.

But we can quit smoking if we follow the following suggested steps:

- If you have a strong willpower, you can just stop smoking, just now, today, because you are aware that smoking is bad for your health and your family is worried about your health as they love you and need you. So just decide to leave smoking and quit it now.

- There are better things to do in life so why spoil your life by smoking which is useless, costly, and injurious to own health.

- If you have tried to quit smoking and failed then try to reduce it. You should change your brand of cigarette. Buy costly cigarettes so that it pinches you financially and have only 15% to 20% of number of cigarettes, that you are smoking today. By adopting this method, you may have a cigarette packet in your pocket, but you are trying to reduce smoking since the brand is costly, which in turn will elevate your prestige among your friends the moment you take out a costly cigarette packet. As you reduce smoking, your smoking urge will also reduce and one day you can just Stop smoking.

- You love your family. You love your parents, your spouse, your children. Every time you smoke in the house, other family members including your children are facing passive smoking, 'which is equally injurious to health'. You should quit smoking for the sake of your family because you love them and you are wasting your hard-earned money.

- You should also quit smoking as smokers are not respected in the society anymore. The smell of cigarette smoking keeps the smokers in one corner in board room, they are sent to a remote corner in the airport for smoking. You are not welcome to smoke in public places. Your family members are no longer comfortable with your company as a smoker. They only tolerate you because they love you.

- Last but not the least, you have struggled a lot to become successful in your career/ life. You must enjoy now and enjoy for a longer period of time. You must help yourself to live longer by adopting good habits and by shedding bad habits like smoking, which you can do using your 'own strong willpower'. Leave smoking now, leave it today, and you will be just fine. Instead have more water, more fruits, and nuts which are healthy and would make you forget SMOKING, WHICH IS AN INJURIOUS HABIT.

- Restrictions imposed by all Govts. of the various countries, the downsizing of Tobacco industry, also tell us to reduce or stop smoking. A step to reduce Tobacco industry is a people's welfare measure. We should watch the bad physical problems the smokers are facing, throughout the world, and learn a lesson out of it and stop smoking.

- Not smoking would also make us a more respectable and more acceptable member of the society, hence we must try to reduce or stop smoking at the earliest to live longer and enjoy this wonderful life, the Gift of God.

How to stop or reduce drinking Alcohol

Drinking hard liquor like Whiskey, Rum, Vodka, etc., or even wine has now become a habit of lot of people in present era.

The young ones are starting to drink in their teens. The teenagers are now getting used to 'Tequila shots', and other liquor brand quite early in age.

The young generation are used to parties, the great source of enjoyment, by drinking liquor and dancing with Jazz or Rock music.

The so-called friends pull other friends to the dancing floor to dance. Some of them drink and influence others to drink. The parties last very long as everyone enjoys such parties and eventually, even non-drinkers are attracted to drinks, thinking they would enjoy more after getting 'a little high', after one/two pegs of Whiskeys / Rums / Vodkas, etc.

Some matured ones/ elders, drink in the parties, etc., as social drinking. They remain sober and normally behave well even after a few drinks, being well educated and respectable elites of the society.

There are others however, who drink very heavily to get 'Kicks' and quite a few of them, lose control of themselves after getting drunk and, at times, misbehave in parties or gatherings, causing unpleasant incidents.

There are few people, who drink every day to enjoy life, but drink heavily as they are not satisfied with one or two or even three large pegs. They keep increasing their quota of pegs for drinking to enjoy the drinks. There are people who consume a full bottle of whiskey every evening, which is extremely harmful for our body in addition to transforming us into an uncivilised social animal who, at times, may commit heinous crimes under the state of utter intoxication, as they are not in their normal senses during this period.

There are also some respectable and sensible people, who consume 6 to 7 pegs of hard drinks a day, in their own home. They behave well and stay normal even after 'good amount of intake of hard drinks'. But they harm their health while enjoying their drink.

We must know that human body's inner lining of gut consists of a single cell layer of intestinal epithelium, through which the hard liquor comes to big intestine, It is dangerous to drink hard liquor at a young age as the intestine is very tender at that age. Hard drink may damage the intestine/liver.

Even at an advanced age, when adults drink heavily, it affects their intestine, liver, kidneys, etc., causing diseases like Liver Cirrhosis, etc.

Enjoy longer, live longer by not drinking or drinking less

We have only one life. we want to live longer for ourselves and our families. The drinks in a small quantity may give us a good feeling, may calm our nerves, and may be enjoyable. Social drinking with one or two pegs, a couple of times a week, say on weekends, can be enjoyable. But over-drinking is bad for our health.

If we use our strong willpower, we can reduce our drinking, if not totally stop drinking.

We must think of enjoying for a longer period and live longer to enjoy our life as we have worked very hard to reach this stage of life which is successful and comfortable.

We should not be foolish enough to give away our most precious and valuable life, just for a bad habit like drinking hard liquor.

We can reduce the intake and still enjoy. People who get drunk in parties, etc., are not respected at all. In fact, they become social outcast because few of them misbehave after heavy drinking. Let us live a healthier life without drinking or less drinking, as drinking cannot reduce our sadness, or frustration, or stress, on the contrary, it increases our trouble including avoidable health problems like Liver Cirrhosis, lack of sleep, etc.

CHAPTER XIII

How to manage our Failure and Success in life

How to manage our failure

"It is fine to celebrate success, but is more important to heed the lessons of failure" – Bill Gates

It is sad, difficult, and demoralizing to fail. May it be an exam, an interview or any project.

One feels worse if one prepares well and yet fail.

Failure is addition to own sadness, mental discomfort, also allows happiness to your competitors or unfriendly people. People who are jealous of you, or who are not happy seeing you successful. People who want to replace you or want to be in the same position you are trying to be. There are lot of unkind and curt people who do not like to or want you to be successful.

If you unfortunately fail, you lose your face in your friend circle, in the society. People start neglecting you and ignoring you.

Even your family suffers from your failure. They also suffer from humiliation like you.

A failure in big project or business, adds on to lot of financial suffering, in addition to emotional distress.

Failure, thus, is a sad incident and is avoidable. But it happens, not once but many times in life. And one may face failure in personal, domestic, as well as professional life.

It is therefore very important to learn lessons from failure and convert failure into success. There is a famous saying that "Failures are pillars for success"

Failure should not deter us but should increase our desire to succeed. The learning from the failures should be the launch pad for success.

History has many examples where kings achieved victory after defeats. Robert Bruce, the king of Scotland, was defeated by the king of England six times. He was hiding in a cave when one day he saw a Spider, trying to climb up but fell six times before it could climb the wall. Robert Bruce learnt a great lesson from the Determined Spider and it's Grit, determination and Resilience to succeed, after repeated failures. Robert Bruce, mastered enough courage, got hold of his men, and fought once again, against the king of England and on the 7th time he was victorious. He defeated the king of England.

Wright Brothers failed in many experiments and many trials before inventing Aeroplanes.

Steps to be taken from failure to success

- Study in great detail about the objective/ goal/ target to be achieved.
- Make a proper plan
- It should be time-bound plan
- It should be a full-proof plan
- Workable
- Unique and innovative
- Within resources available

- Practice the procedure many times to perfect the effort.
- See what was lacking in the effort when the previous attempt failed.
- Rectify the processes that were responsible for failures like lack of practice, lack of resources, any health-related issues, any financial issue, any knowledge or expertise related, technical or legal issue.
- Rectify the flaws in execution procedure.
- Try to innovate a new plan of execution which would have better chance to succeed. British army 'Squares' retaliated Napoleon's mighty cavalry during the battle of Waterloo, which was such an innovative military step.

We may be able to innovate some unique steps to convert failure into success.

Lt .Gen. William Slim, a British General of Allied Force, located in India, converted his defeat into victory in battle of Burma against the mighty Japanese army, in WW II. Burma is now known to be Myanmar.

Gen. Slim's Army, was not trained in jungle warfare and could not put up a good fight against the Japanese Army initially which advanced till Kohima and Imphal, located on the Indian Border in the East. He then trained his army in the hills and forests of East India. Trained, Equipped, and organized his formations as the Army Commander of 14th Army

Lt. Gen. Slim's Army achieved great victory against mighty Japanese Army and liberated Myanmar from the Japanese Army , during World War-II. It was an ideal example of turning Defeat into Victory.

He became a Field Marshal (FM) and he wrote his famous book, "Defeat into Victory", writing about his own experience of detailed measures and preparation he undertook to defeat mighty and gritty Japanese Army, converting his defeat into victory, a very important part of World War II from 1942 to 1945 and success of Allied Forces in the East.

How to manage our success

It is extremely important to understand the meaning of success and manage the effects of success. We all want to be successful in every sphere of our life, i.e., in exams in the schools or colleges, in job interviews, in our all projects in the professional life etc.

Sometimes success comes easily and sometimes success comes after a lot of effort.

But success is a very enjoyable experience. We want to celebrate our success, as success gives us lots of satisfaction, makes us and family members happy, makes us feel rewarded, and gives a tremendous boost to our confidence.

But it is very important to analyse the meaning of success. It is the achievement of our effort to secure our objective, our goal. But there will be bigger goals, bigger and higher objectives in our life. If we are successful in our exams in school, we must continue our good effort to be successful in the college and in professional life and so on, in future as well.

So we must understand that success, in addition to giving us joy, has also warned us of new challenges and these are as follows:-

- 'Success is 1% of inspiration and 99% of perspiration', as said by Thomas Edison. So, the hard work should never stop.

- Enjoy or celebrate success within limits and in a low scale so that "you do not show off" much as the next test, next hurdle, next goal may be much more tough to achieve.

- Success gives confidence but you should not become over-confident because over-confidence may make you excited and careless to commit mistakes which may lead to failure.

"Success is not only about having more money and a higher social status. Success also manifests in being less stressed, less worried and more peaceful and happy", said Remez Sasson, a great writer.

"Success is journey, not a destination. The doing is often more important that the outcome" – said Arthur Ashe Jr, the great Tennis Player of US.

- We need success for all objectives or goals of life, hence enjoy the present success but prepare harder for future objectives.
- Being complacent is detrimental to success.

Adopt excellence as the quality for performance. The habit of performing well would ensure success.

- The best way to compete with the known or unknown competitors is to "RAISE OWN BAR' during preparation, continuously.
- Keep your goals and objectives in your mind and prepare for success silently, without any publicity or exhibition of your strength.
- Being humble and grounded yet determined would always help you to become successful.
- Always consider your competitors and opponents more intelligent and resourceful and powerful. This would elevate your level of preparation for success.

- Most important thing is that no one can always be successful. You may prepare very hard but the element of luck also plays a big role in our life and we may not be lucky always. So we must learn to tackle failure in a very matured way and move ahead with the learning from failure to success and learn to enjoy our success without showing off and continue to prepare hard for a Greater Success.

CHAPTER XIV

We have only one Life and it must be a Happy Life.

We must plan to have a successful and happy life. We work very hard throughout our life to be successful and respected in the society and to enjoy the fruits of our hard work in this life. We try very hard to make our parents and near and dear ones proud of us.

But we must also ensure we have a happy life. The life, whatever way we may plan, would have ups & downs, failure and success, bad days and good days. But there are certain things, if we follow, would make our life, a happy life.

What is Happiness

Happiness is a state of mind. We should keep our mind happy with doing good deeds.

Follow ethics, honesty, rules and laws always. An honest man who follows ethics, rules, laws is always a happy man.

A person who follows unethical means, does not follow rules & laws, may benefit for a short time but he remains always worried to be caught by the authorities. He remains restless, whereas a person who follows ethics, rules, and laws has nothing to fear as he has not done anything unethical or unlawful. He remains peaceful and happy.

Prepare hard to achieve success but embrace failure with equal warmth. We can try to achieve success but, at times, things do not happen the way we want and we may fail to qualify, to get selected, or to succeed. We should try to move ahead without being unhappy with the result.

Give back to the society. The society and the people of the society help us in many ways, both directly and indirectly. It is therefore our duty to help the society, its needy people, sick people, and poor people in whatever way we can.

There are many examples like Florence Nightingale, Mother Teresa, Mr. Warren Buffet, and Mr. Bill Gates who have helped the people of the society and some of them are still helping the people of the society, irrespective of their country, religion, caste, greed and colour. Giving back to the society gives us ultimate happiness.

Simple tips to make our life happy

- Never compare yourself with others. You have your qualities, your values, you are what you are, and you will get what you are destined to get, with all your sincere efforts. Be happy what you are today and in whatever way you are. Don't be unhappy comparing yourself with so called more successful people, because who knows, you may be happier than them.

- Forget the past. The failure of past, the rejections of past, regarding how you very narrowly missed an opportunity to change your life. Remembering the failed attempts of past would be very painful, and would invariably make you more unhappy. Forget the past, think of present time and plan for future, and hope for the best.

- Try to make an unhappy man happy by helping a needy, sick and poor person.

- Appreciate what you have, love them, and care for them. Every field at a distance looks greener but in reality, it may not be so. Be happy with what you got and what you have. God always gives us more than we deserve. Appreciate what you have as God's blessings, or else you may lose this also if you neglect what you have.

- Don't envy anyone, everyone gets what he deserves, It is of no use being jealous of others. We should try hard in an appropriate way to change, and elevate our life.

- Learn to forget and forgive. Try to inculcate the habit of forgetting and forgiving. There will be a lot of instances where people will ill treat you, misbehave with you and even try to cheat you. Forgetting and forgiving people is an easier solution to get peace of mind and happiness or else such incidents and such people would keep bothering you and disturbing you throughout your life. Hatred increases hatred. Taking revenge in no solution to a problem. Solving a problem with a mutually agreed, respectable, and long-term peaceful solution would be ideal.

How to build a strong personality.

A person should be strong to face the challenges of the present world. The modern world needs qualities of a person which can tackle traditional values, modern technology, and complex human behaviour. The modern era has a mix culture. The people of most of the countries are mix of various cultures. If the husband is a British, the wife may be a German, if the father is a Hindu, the mother could be Buddhist, etc.

The young generation, who are technologically advanced, are struggling to follow or even believe in the values they were taught in the younger days by the parents, schools, and colleges. As they grow up, they are exposed to the world which may have different values, culture, norms, etc.

Today's generation is very enlightened, well aware of things, are much more mature than their grandparents and parents in their age.

Today's generation, though very smart, knowledgeable and progressive, face social challenges like excessive competition in their academic career, professional career, teenage pregnancy, drugs, relationship, etc. Though their lives are comfortable as compared to their previous generation, because of more discoveries, inventions and technological advancement, they are emotionally and physically weak. Present generation must build their personality very strong on the following aspects:

1. Mental

2. Physical

3. Emotional

It is very important to develop mental strength. Today's generation is always over stressed because of the studies, pressure to excel in career, competition etc.

Since all parents want their children to do well in life, there is a tremendous competition among the young children/students. Every year, few students, commit suicide, as they cannot cope up with the pressure.

We have only one life and surviving in the life and making it a pleasurable journey should be our aim. Parent's aim and children's aim must be respected, but not at the cost of one's life. We must make our children mentally strong enough to face the challenges of life including studies, career, and so on. At no stage, a life can be sacrificed for academic or professional career. Parents must observe the children's behaviour and communicate with them more frequently, and tell them that their lives are most important, their failure or success, notwithstanding.

Children should be taught to see big dreams, but it should be as per his/her choice, his/her liking and most importantly as per his/her capacity. They should not be pushed to select a career, just because some relative's children, or neighbour children have chosen.

Parents must understand that a child can excel in any field. There are various examples before us like Shakespeare, Einstein, John Kennedy, Rabindranath Tagore, Beethoven, Mozart, Isaac Newton, Adin Smith, Abraham Lincoln, Mahatma Gandhi, Nelson Mandela, Van Gogh, Michael Angelo, Leonardo Da Vinci, Words Worth, Charles Dickens, and many more. A child can choose any line and fulfil his/her dream. He/she does not have to follow or copy anyone. He may appreciate someone or their ideas, but should work hard in his chosen field to be successful. Success is also a comparative term. A child should be allowed to do what he likes to do, or is interested to do so that he can be happy. There are many options available for a child at present.

"Children must be taught how to think, not what to think." Said Margaret Mead, which is so important for a child's growth.

Mental Strength

A child should not be allowed to be 'mentally tired'. He may be physically tired for chasing his dream but if he gets mentally tired, then that will be dangerous, as it may lead to frustration, depression and sleepless nights, etc., hence must be avoided.

Mental strength is also very important as we reach senior level as we would be working with equally qualified as well as experienced people. We would be interacting with the competitors at the highest level if we are the CEOs, and mental strength is extremely important at this stage, for negotiations, convincing the competitors, representing own organization well and to its advantage.

Physical strength

It is very important for a person to be physically fit. Only a physically fit person can be mentally fit.

Today's generations are privileged to have all the technical gadgets like mobile, computer, cars, motorcycles, internet with various apps etc. These are very good for comfortable life but these items/facilities have made us home bound, chair bound and less physically active.

Today's children play football on TV, they are addicted to mobiles and are continuously engaged with internet/computers. They are not playing physical/games like Football, Basket Ball, Volley Ball, Hockey, Boxing, etc., that often, hence most of them are physically weak.

They fall sick often as they are under huge pressure of studies, modern lifestyle like travelling, going for parties, clubs, consumption of excess food, drinks, etc. Quite a lot of them smoke which reduces the energy level of a person.

One must remember that remaining healthy is the top most priority of our life. If we are not healthy, we cannot enjoy our life. We may be rich, but a physically weak person cannot even eat properly, cannot travel to places one would like to visit, cannot attend regular activities which his friends would be able to attend, like college parties, fresher's parties, graduation ceremonies, etc.

With the advanced medical treatments, Medicines, etc., our lifespan is increasing. A lot of people are now living beyond 80's. One has to be very careful from the childhood to remain physically fit to enjoy a long life.

A physically fit person can also work for a long time. The retirement age of all most all countries are increasing to 65-70 years. One must remain physically fit to even work for longer period so that even at the age of 60-70 he is fit enough to work and remain engaged positively which also keeps a person healthy & happy.

Emotional Strength

In present scenario, emotional strength of a person has become very important. Today's generations need to be stronger emotionally.

The joint family system has perished. We have a small family now. Mom, dad, and one child, at most 2 children. The children are most precious to any parents. Children are therefore pampered. They get everything they want, easily.

A child handles a tablet when he is just 2 years old, a mobile phone from 5 years, has car as a teenager, travels abroad as a child during his school holidays. He gets everything he wants and becomes pampered and eventually, in some cases, spoilt. He, therefore, is not used to listening to no, not available, etc., but the real life is totally different. People and the world may not care who he is, hence he gets frustrated when he does not get something which he wants, or when he faces failure or rejection in life. Very recently in Mumbai, India, a young boy jumped in the sea from a bridge and died because he found out that his girlfriend was dating another boy. The deceased was the only child of his parents. With his untimely demise, his dreams, his parent's dreams, and his parents were all shattered.

He was emotionally so weak that he did not think about his parents at all before taking this drastic decision to end life.

He was also not mature or smart enough to understand that if his girlfriend was dating some other boy, she did not deserve him or he should have been smart enough to move on and not finish his own life, which did not just belong to him but it also belonged to his parents and the society. How about his responsibilities towards his old parents and the society which gave him so much all these years? Being emotionally strong is therefore extremely important.

Emotional Quotient(EQ), is an extremely good quality of a person in today's world, especially in our Professional Career.

Be Smart not to lose any opportunity coming your way.

In our life, it is seldom that we get an opportunity to do something which may change our life forever. Many of us do not understand it, many of us ignore it, not knowing the value of the opportunity and repent later on.

On the contrary, there are people who grab the opportunity and work hard to take advantage of it and get tremendous success in their lives later.

Opportunity comes but once, and we should be smart enough, alert enough, and sensible enough to take advantage of it and use it to our advantage.

Opportunities are God sent and we must not miss these and repent throughout our life for missing such opportunities.

Relation between Materialism and Happiness

In Economics we study about Propensity to Consume. There is average propensity to consume, the urge of a consumer to consume over the total income and there is Marginal Propensity to Consume, the urge of a consumer to increase consumption over a marginal increase of income, i.e., over more disposable income.

More disposable income drives the consumer to buy more items, which they do not have, The normal psychology of an average consumer is to watch others, neighbours, friends, etc., and buy those items which others have and he does not have. It is basically to remove the feeling of inferiority complex that one suffers from. If a friend has 65" TV and himself has a 32" TV, if the friend has Mercedes car and he has a Honda City and things like that the urge of buying more items grows as the disposable income grows. The urge of purchasing grows from less costly items to costlier items, from items of basic necessity to luxury items, from TV, washing machine, cars to flats, bungalows and so on.

Materialism is an addiction. It drives consumers crazy and leads them to buy items even beyond their financial limits.

People use multiple credit cards, savings to buy items, basically to show off to their friends and neighbours that they are now doing financially well. Such unwarranted and avoidable expenditure leads the consumers to debt and endless financial stress.

In situation like Covid-19 epidemic, when a lot of people lost their jobs throughout the world, people got into debt trap and faced a very tough financial situation. Especially in the families where both the husband and wife lost their jobs. It was very difficult to run the family and pay EMIs for car, flats etc., which caused a lot of financial stress.

The materialism therefore, has to be very carefully handled and monitored as the excess of materialism may lead to lot of financial stress and mental stress.

A lot of well-known business men have committed suicide for taking excessive loan for their business as the EMIs could not be paid on time due to situation like Covid-19, or global economic meltdown at times. Excessive materialism therefore leads to a lot of unhappiness. It is better to live within our own means, avoiding loans and credit cards and financial misery.

Materialism, in fact makes man unhappy, as his unlimited demands never ends and he chases happiness and better status in the society by acquiring various goods , which eventually , leads him to financial problems and unhappiness.

Role of spirituality in our life

Spirituality is an individual divine thought process that enables a person to pray to God, become a simple, humble, and empathic person who wants to help all other people who need help, irrespective of their religion, country, culture, and language.

For a spiritual person the entire world is his family.

A spiritual person has following good qualities:

- He is God-fearing
- He is honest
- He is simple
- He is helpful to all
- He thinks beyond religion, country, culture, and language.
- He is friendly and helpful to all
- He always thinks positive and avoids argument with anyone.
- He is extremely mature, kind, and big-hearted.

- He believes in forgetting and forgiving
- He believes in God, the ultimate divine power, who blesses us, helps us all the time. He respects his own God as per his religion and respects every other religion and their Gods.
- A spiritual person avoids any bad habits.
- He is trustworthy and respectable.
- He respects humanity, going beyond the religion.
- He is humble and respected for his humility.
- Spirituality in our personal, domestic, and also in our professional life is extremely important as it saves us, and discourages us from doing anything wrong, harming someone, and cheating someone or any organization.

Spiritual Quotient (SQ) is one of the greatest qualities required in higher professional level as it ensures good governance in an organization, as a spiritual man is unbiased, impartial, matured, decent, empathetic and honest.

Senior executives/ Leaders, if spiritual, are empathetic, grounded, and approachable which solves a lot of complex cases in any organization. It also helps in senior level in professional dealings as spiritual people are honest in their dealings which would serve the organizational interest well.

Spirituality is a unique quality of a person. A person who follows spirituality rises beyond religion. he may continue to follow his own religious beliefs, customs, and practices but he would be mature enough to accommodate others from other religions. He would respect other religions and try to help people in addition to his own religion and community.

A spiritual person loves everyone, considers the entire world as his own home, considers everyone of this world as his own, hence he extends his helping hand to everyone. He is a kind, broad-minded person with liberal thoughts. He believes in no discrimination, and is fair to all.

E.g. Warren Buffett, and Bill Gate have pledged to give away their entire life's saving and wealth for the help of the poor, needy, and sick of the world for the welfare of the people as well as for future generation of the world. They contribute to help the world in global warming, poverty, healthcare, agriculture, solar power, alternative energy to reduce carbon emissions and so on. They want to help the entire world and not only US, their own country.

Need of Spiritual Quotient, at Senior Level

Spirituality and Spiritual Quotient (SQ) have become very important at decision making level that is senior level.

Since spiritual people are God-fearing, follow ethics, rules, laws, they are honest and trust worthy.

At the senior level, a person has to take various decisions on behalf of the organization.

A corrupt person may get engaged in Insider Trading or taking decision keeping in view of his own self-interest.

A person with proper spiritual quotient would refrain from taking any such decisions, to benefit his or her family, etc.

A person with good SQ would also behave well with his staff and colleagues as people at senior position enjoy a lot of power. They decide not only organization's future but also fate of its people. SQ would automatically ensure proper behaviour of senior professionals.

Effect of Spiritual Poverty at Senior Level

It is extremely important for the people at senior level to be spiritually sound. Spiritual Poverty or lack of spirituality at the senior level, can be very harmful and even disastrous for self and the organization they lead.

Spiritual poverty would have negative affect in the following:

- Inter personal relationships
- Apt and objective decision making
- Own honesty and integrity
- Unsympathetic decisions which may create employee's anger and attrition of talents.
- Lack of matured and unbiased behaviour, which are extremely important for man management.

At the senior level when you are interacting with other senior executives, senior colleagues, senior officials and counterparts of other organizations, your behaviour, attitude, and language are very important. Spiritual poverty can make a person arrogant, egoistic, and even at times, impolite. All these eventually can affect the well-being of the organization. This kind of behaviour may discourage and demotivate own colleagues and employees as well as suppliers, contractors, dealers, etc., which would hamper the growth of the organization.

The additional Mile that you will have to travel to remain ahead of others

We have only one life and we have to survive and survive well. We try to be successful and achieve our goal over life's objectives. We are in the race with others and we swim along with the rest of the crowd, individually though, maintaining secretly, our ambition, our own goal. People who follow others, especially the successful ones, may cross the finishing line of the so-called success line. They may achieve a comfortable life and give comfort to his family and near and dear ones.

But the finishing line of success is different for different people. It is your own ambition, own target, own goal that drives you to achieve greater success than others.

And that is why we have to travel an Extra or Additional Mile to achieve that more difficult goal, to achieve more than others, to fulfil our special Dream which can help the world like Einstein, Newton, James Watt, Adam Smith, John Keynes, and Steve Jobs did.

What does it involve?

1. Ambition

a) To achieve greater heights in life, career, & profession, we must have an ambition to achieve something greater.

b) An urge to help the society, the people of the world, the desire to give back to the society.

2. Hard work: Unobserved continued hard work, a resilient mindset, and tenacity to accomplish the goal, the target.

3. Result: Own satisfaction, own pride but benefit of the world, and its people in terms of facilities, employment and benefits. People of the world must be benefited by our achievement our innovation our discoveries.

4. Continuous self-motivation: It is very important to continuously motivate ourselves to work hard and excel in our lives. Self-motivation inspires us and turns the failures into success.

The additional or extra mile is not everyone's cup of tea. The great leaders in military, politics, business, academics, science, etc., have achieved it after a lot of hard work, preparation, and sacrifice. But traveling an extra mile puts us above the rest as it enables us to achieve greater results. The journey of the extra mile is what makes us legends to be emulated by many in future.

CHAPTER XV

A Suggested Road Map for Good Life

We have only one life and our aim should be to spend a good life, so that there are no regrets when the life ends eventually.

Some Important Steps To Be Followed To Achieve A Good Life

a) Ethics

Ethics, honesty, and integrity are extremely important qualities in today's global world.

b) Excellence

The world is heartless, rude, and a merciless battle-field. Only the best would survive the competitions. Hence, excellence must be our motto. We must be the best in whatever we do. We must prepare hard, be resilient, and be determined to achieve our goal.

c) Health

We must be careful about our health, we must do regular physical excuse but not overdo it, to keep ourselves physically fit. We must watch our diet and avoid unhealthy food and harmful habits.

d) Happiness

We must learn to be happy in our life. Life is short but it should be happy. A rich man may be unhappy and poor man may be happy. A professionally successful man may be unhappy and a less successful man may be happy. Happiness is a state of mind. We should be happy with small achievements, small day to day activities, family functions, religious celebrations like Diwali, Christmas, Eid, etc. We must know that our families, and children give us maximum happiness. We should celebrate every occasion, without waiting for a big event or big achievement. Life is short and uncertain, remaining happy therefore, is our prerogative. But we must do good deeds and pray to God, whenever we get the time, to get his Blessings. God's Blessings create Miracles.

Be Unique, be Different, Nothing is free in this world (Said The Famous, Mr. Jack Ma, Chairman of Alibaba)

If you want to be successful, you have to pay the price. Nothing is free.

The idea which everyone likes or thinks to be good is rubbish because everyone thinks it is good, hence it won't work.

But if there is an idea which is very difficult, almost impossible to achieve, should be considered as it is done differently and if done with quality, this idea would succeed. If it is a difficult objective, and not everyone's 'cup of tea', hence must be tried out.

We should therefore be different, i**nnovative** and ready to work hard to achieve our goal, which must be a difficult one, to become successful in life.

Learn Soft Skills To Survive

Communication skills

The most important quality of a person nowadays is his communication skills. It is a two-way process; hence it is extremely important that opposite side should hear us properly, understand us properly so that he/she can communicate properly with us.

Communication can be verbal, written, and when in close proximity, non-verbal. It should be clear, short, in simple language which both partners understand, should be decent polite and civilized. It is very important for our day to day function in domestic, personal and professional life. It is a great quality to influence people and all great leaders were eloquent speakers. Learning and mastering communication skills, therefore, is a very important asset in modern era.

Leadership

There are two categories of people in this world one category consists of leaders and the other category consists of the led.

We are all born with almost same qualities but few of us inculcate, develop, and learn few qualities which take them ahead of the others. They then lead the group, and others simply follow. We all know and read about the qualities of leaders. We know that leaders nowadays are made and very few are born leaders. Apart from descendants of the kings and Queens, who are very few at present, the leaders are made because of their great qualities. Abraham Lincoln, Mahatma Gandhi, Nelson Mandela are few such examples. Jack Welch, Steve Jobs are other examples in the corporate world.

The important qualities of a leader at present are:

Courage, honesty, vision, being tech savvy, empathetic, inter-personal relationship, servanthood, adaptability, keen learner, apt qualifications, and skills, maturity, excellent communication skills, physical, emotional and mental fitness, broad mindedness and spirituality.

Today's leaders are global leaders as the world has become a global village. A leader has to lead people of multiple countries, religion, culture, languages region etc.

Today's leader must be highly qualified, innovative, accommodative, and adaptive. He must be respected for his dealings and qualities, and contributions to the organization which will make him an acceptable and loved by his people.

Types of Leaderships

There are various types of leaderships that we are already aware of, some of the important ones are mentioned below:

1. Autocratic

2. Democratic

3. Paternalistic

Few more well-known and appreciated types of leadership are:

1. Transactional and Transformational

2. Charismatic

3. Visionary

But in present era we must also learn following leadership skills

- Role of emotional intelligence in leadership
- Maxwell's 5 level of leadership
- Leadership in era of Artificial Intelligence

- Global leadership

Problem solving skills

Problem solving has become a quality that is greatly appreciated now. Every organization wants a problem solver. Problem solving is quality which can be inculcated by learning, and following these skills:

- Develop an eye for details
- Develop analytical skills
- Try to reach the roots of a problem
- Think out of box for the solution
- Be innovative
- Try to understand the problem properly
- Find a permanent solution and not a temporary one.
- Be impartial and unbiased
- Give a practical, realistic, and honest solution
- An ethical, honest, impartial, and permanent solution will always be respected and accepted.

Patience

Patience in a person is a very important and rare quality. It is a winning quality in a person. A person with patience wins many 'battles' as the opponent gets tired, irritated, and often loses mental balance.

Patience, as a quality, is important in our personal, domestic, and professional life. A person with patience, deals with problems in a different way, with his calmness and composure. A patient person remains dignified, and respectable to deal with any situation rather than losing his cool or temper. He listens to the other party patiently and convinces him with suitable and win-win solution. The other party listens to him as he is patient, calm, and respectful and tried to solve the issue with his patience and calmness.

Confidence

Confidence of person keeps him ahead of others. A confident person knows his job and performs better than others.

To earn confidence however one has to do the following:

a) Prepare well for the task/ job/ assignment

b) Work harder than others to feel confident to perform better

c) Raise your own bar of efficiency to be better than the competitors

d) Should not show-off but prepare silently having more practice, for gaining confidence

e) Avoid being proud or over-confident, which might spoil the performance

f) Success and confidence should be smartly used for achieving more success

Empathy

As human resource management has become very important now, the leaders should be empathetic, they must have empathy, i.e., be able to put themselves in the shoes of others to understand their problems, before taking a decision.

The decisions of an empathetic leaders is often accepted and appreciated by the employees. A lot of critical issue can be solved by being empathetic, as an empathetic leader has greater influence on the workforce.

All of us therefore should understand the importance of empathy which is a very essential quality of a leader.

Flexibility

All of us must learn to be flexible in our approach, may it be personal front, domestic front, or even professional front. Rigidity spoils things, rigidity blocks our mind and minimizes our logic. We must appreciate criticism and be flexible to change our thought process. Sycophancy ultimately, is dangerous and may lead us to wrong ends.

We should be open to discuss the matter with the colleagues which may even give us a better solution.

Flexibility needs power of tolerance, a big and honest heart, and a resilient mind. The quality of flexibility enhances the chances of success.

Flexibility is very important to manage a team.

Adaptability to change

Change, in our life, is a constant phenomenon. Due to advanced technology, change is taking place in every sphere of life.

Adaptability to change is considered a great quality in a person now as we are now living in VUCA environment, which is volatile, uncertain, complex and ambiguous, and at times even chaotic.

Adaptability to change enables us to survive in new environment with new technology and changed atmosphere.

The era of Artificial Intelligence is going to revolutionize and change the entire world. Adaptability will help us to learn new skills, adopt new norms and remain relevant and useful to a new set-up.

Team Man

"If you want to go fast, go alone, but if you can want to go far, go along with others". It is very important to be a Team Man, in present era. With more and more flat organizations, people are working in smaller teams. In the global business, which is spreading over the entire world, one has to be team man, as small teams operate, in various parts of the world.

One has to work with people of multiple culture, multiple religion, languages, and countries. Only a team man, who understand and can adjust with his colleagues, will survive. Hence, all of us must be a team man or learn to be a team man to survive in any organization.

Decision Making

The decision-making ability is a very important quality of a person in his personal life, domestic life, and professional life. It's a good quality of a leader.

Decision making needs planning, preparation, getting into details, and thinking of repercussion after the decision has been made.

Decisiveness is a great quality of a person and that of a leader. In the professional field at times harsh decisions have to be taken in the interest of the organization. Few leaders may hesitate or delay the decision hurting the organization even more. A good leader takes the proper decision when needed and has the guts to face it. He, however, has to do the homework. The decision should be goal-oriented, empathetic, keeping in view the organization's goal as well as the welfare of the its people.

Social Skills

Social skills are very important in present era. Knowing your people and keeping good relation with them is extremely important for the organization. An organization is managed by men, machine, money and technology. Out of all these ingredients men are the most important as they manage the other three ingredients. Social skills and inter personal relationships have become very important as we deal with educated and skilled knowledge workers.

It is also important as we work and manage a multicultural, multilingual, multi religious works force spread over the entire world.

Social skills depend on the following aspects:

Knowing the people

Respecting them their culture, origin, language, religion, and lifestyle

Being empathetic and humble

Following ethics and being unbiased

Good Etiquette

Etiquette is code of conduct and set of rules in the society that are required for positive human interactions, It is like law. E.g. Dress code, Soft skills, Etiquette at work.

Mannerism

Mannerism is behaviour that reflects a person's attitude, behaviour that we practice to follow etiquette.

E.g.

- Telephone Manners: To be polite, Lower tone, Happy sounding and Respectful
- Verbal and Written communications must be polite and respectful
- Conversations should be Pleasant
- Language must be polite and decent.

Decent Behaviour

Be polite, helpful, decent, don't be rude, be kind, be positive, be cooperative, respect other's privacy, be pleasant and behave well.

Skills and good practices to keep the life on track

1. We have only one life, and it cannot be wasted. One has to plan his/her life well to travel the journey well, enjoy it, achieve the goals planned for and keep the memorable footprints for others to remember us and follow us in future. This would keep us alive long after we are gone, for example, Mahatma Gandhi, Abraham Lincoln, Late Lata Mangeshkar- the Great Indian Singer, Sir Don Bradman- the Australian Cricketer, Pele- the Great footballer, Albert Einstein- the scientist, Rabindranath Tagore- the poet, William Shakespeare- the writer, etc.

2. Dream big and shape yourself. We have to dream big to achieve something spectacular, to become successful in life.

If we dream big, we will start working for it, prepare hard to achieve our goals. Those of us who do not dream big or do not dream at all to do well in life, lead a mediocre life and struggle throughout life, remaining merely passenger. The near and dear ones including the family, parents also suffer because of the lackadaisical attitude of these people towards life.

3. Never forget the value of your parents. They are your friends forever. Today you need them, tomorrow they may need you, please remember that.

4. Educate your mind and heart both. "Educating the mind and heart without educating the heart is no education at all" – Aristotle

It is extremely important that we educate our mind and heart both. Only then we will be able to respect people, tolerate people, and love people irrespective of cast, creed, religion, region, colour, culture, language.

This quality is extremely important to become a good international citizen. The Globalization needs an international approach, mindset, attitude, and liberal, as well as broadminded nature.

Educating mind and heart would help us achieve that. It avoids any kind of discrimination, promotes brotherhood, and helps in achieving spirituality.

5. Avoid shortcuts in life. It is a human nature to have shortcuts. We take shortcuts to save time, to get success, to impress others to manipulate our financial state to overtake our colleagues in professional life and so on. But invariably the so-called shortcut leads us to long journey.

E.g. A boy trying to cross a busy road avoiding the over bridge meant for the same purpose, may meet with an avoidable accident.

A student using unfair means to get good marks in an exam, getting caught by the invigilator, and getting debarred from the exam.

It is therefore very important to teach children to avoid any kind of shortcuts in life, which ultimately saves time, money and earns respect and dignity of a person.

Role of love, lust, laughter and leisure in our life

Love

True love is a total surrender to the partner because we love her/him with all our heart, brain, and mind.

We can do anything for the partner because even she/he loves us that much, maybe even more.

Take the example of the wives of India. A girl gets married to person, comes along with him, 1000 of Kms away, leaving her home, parents, brothers, sisters, relations and friends.

She surrenders herself completely to the husband, in some cases, a totally unknown person and his family. Since she loves him, and got even married to him, she comes with him to his house, try to keep him and his family happy in every way. Her sincerity, dedication, her caring, loving nature, change the husband's life to a better life, and gives real happiness. She becomes the pivot of his family, mother of his children. His world changes for happy days forever, because of her love.

If we, do not surrender, ourselves also, to get completely immersed in her love, then our love would be incomplete. Sacrifice, surrender and trust are extremely important in love.

Love in Modern times

The word love in modern times, in times of high technology and economic independence, however is quite different.

People have become very materialistic and true love, genuine love, innocent love has taken a back seat.

Nowadays people consider various matrix before falling in love or expressing their love.

But, alas, as the material world changes, as economic condition changes, as the so-called 'statues of people' changes, love also changes. It unfortunately evaporates at times, as it is based on materialistic success or failure.

Let us try to love by our heart and not our calculative brain or else there will never be true love.

Lust

Lust is a craving to have something. Lust makes a person crazy to have something that he is so keen to have. It also means strong desire to have sex, with someone who may not be interested and have it forcefully.

Lust is a strong emotional expression of animals including human beings. It also turns a human being into animal as he does things, due to lust or effect of lust in his mind, which may be, at times, prove to be harmful for others or done with or without the consent of another person. Rape is an ideal example of lust where a man forces a female for sex.

Lust may make a person crazy to do other improper things, leading to heinous crimes e.g. rape and murder of a victim. Lust makes a man insane, crazy, ruthless and dangerous. A normal man, can become a criminal, due to lust. Lust though at times, may be a culminating effect of love, is a negative expression of emotion and must be controlled.

A person with education and maturity may be able to control lust, which would ensure his respect and dignity.

Lust, therefore, falls short of love which is based on sacrifice, surrender, and well-being of opposite partner with whom we are in love as we want to see our partner happy at all cost. Lust on the other hand is an arrogant desire to make us happy to acquire or have something, even forcibly, if needed, to fulfil our inner desire to get or have something that we crave to get even, at times, without the consent of the partner.

Laughter

Laughter is an essential and natural expression of happiness. We smile when we are happy, we laugh when we are very happy. Laughter is a positive reaction of our emotional outburst. If we like a joke we laugh aloud. When we get a pleasant surprise by someone, very dear one, coming to our home, suddenly, we welcome him with a smile. When we get good news like passing in exam or in an important job interview, we feel happy and we laugh and enjoy the moment. When we read something funny in a book we may laugh aloud, when we see something funny in a movie, we laugh aloud.

Laughter is a very healthy physical gesture, it is good for lungs, it is healthy. It makes the muscles and nerves of the face work, which is good for face muscles and the health.

Our laughter may make others, near us laugh as well, which is a friendly gesture.

Laughter is especially important for senior citizen, as people forget to smile, leave alone laugh, at advanced age. So whenever it is possible, one should laugh and if possible laugh aloud ,which is good for lungs, heart and our body.

In the modern era, where families are small, children, quite often, study abroad or work somewhere else, parents and elders are lonely. The chances of laughter are very less.

The changing advance technologies/ Gadgets also keep us busy with all technical gadgets. People hardly meet friends and in advanced age, we hardly move out. The chances of laughter reduce to a great extent.

There are however some laughter classes / gatherings in some parks or clubs, in the early morning. People should take advantage of that and laugh and laugh louder whenever possible.

It is our life, let us enjoy it.

Leisure

Leisure is the free time when people spend time, doing what they want to do, away from everyday responsibilities from official work or domestic tasks. Leisure is the time to Rest, Relax and Enjoy Life. Leisure is not working to earn money, Leisure is to recharge our batteries, do things we would love to do and enjoy the time so that we go back to work fresh and more energetic.

People normally do things of their interest during leisure like follow hobbies or play some games, or do things which is self-entertaining, enjoyable and relaxing.

Leisure is our own time, there is no time bound or compulsive, dedicated agenda. It is what we want to do.

Understood that leisure time is limited in this task oriented, competitive, fastmoving world. We all have to work to survive, we all have to earn our livelihood and work hard to be comfortable and to make our family comfortable, but our body and mind need some rest. Even a good machine may fail if not maintained well or rested periodically.

We, human beings, though very busy in our day to day activities, must rest sometimes, giving our body, mind the brain, some rest.

Leisure is therefore very important so that we can get some rest, mentally and physically, and return fresh for work.

In present era, a lot of people are having health problem at young age. The life is very taxing, long office hours, huge responsibilities, meeting the deadlines / targets, keep us very busy, especially at senior level. Lot of young CEO's are suffering from various health issues because of the stress.

Times for leisure at regular intervals are very important for a long journey, which rejuvenates us and keeps us happy, healthy and energetic.

Leisure time should be planned by everyone well in advance so that neither the work, nor the health suffers.

We can work if we survive.

Without periodical leisure, one cannot bear the work load/ responsibilities for a long time.

Leisure also allows the family members and children, sometime, to be with us which is quite rare now a days because of everyone's busy schedule. Leisure is, therefore, a welcome change, for the family members also, which everyone needs.

CHAPTER XVI

Value of Time and Time Management

The importance of Time in our life.

The costliest thing we have in our life is 'TIME'. The second or minute or hour or the day, just gone, will never come back. No one, with any amount of money, or power can get this time back.

Yet most of us do not really understand the importance of time management. If we learn to manage the time, we would be able to utilize the time properly and not waste it.

In one of the previous chapters, we have discussed about the importance of the Decider Decade, that proper utilization and planning of a youth's career and upbringing from age of 13/14 to 23/24, is most crucial for proper development of his life.

Time management teaches us to get up early in the morning and thereby gain 2/3 hours in a day of 24 hours. There are people who get up at 8 or 9 am or 10 am. They then lose 2 or 3 costly hours of the day, when they could do few important things, like doing physical exercise or study, planning for day, etc. The concentration level is very high in the early morning hence anything done in the early morning, remains useful and fruitful.

If we can get up at 5.00 am or 5.30 am, we can plan our entire day's work properly.

The fresh air in the early morning, is not only healthy but also generates lot of positivity. Our body and mind become fresh, active and joyful. Morning workouts are always good as the body is more energetic after the night's rest.

The morning hours are the best in this beautiful world, created by the God.

The fresh air, the dews on the green grass, the fresh blossoming flowers, the trees with leaves of various shades of colours, the smiling friends and their softly spoken 'good morning', together create a beautiful day. The beautiful nature, the birds, the blue sky, the crimson coloured rising sun, starts, yet another magnificent day. And only those who are lucky enough to enjoy all of these, are the ones who get up early every day. It is a beautiful experience which stays in our mind, the entire day.

Getting up early in the morning enables us to plan for the entire day. Especially when a person reaches senior position in an organization or one has big business/industry running, he has a lot of complex issues in his mind and head.

Early morning hours can help us to think about the work in hand and allow us to think to find solutions and plan for the day ahead.

Time Management in simple words is the process of organizing and planning how to divide our time between different activities, allowing them Proper Priority.

This enables us to give priority to the more important work, to finish the work in better time frame and do the less important work, later.

This also helps us to get more things done in less time since things have been planned before.

Planning and finishing the tasks, in hand, on time is important to get rid of the pressure and tension, which invariably grows if things are not planned well and also not done on time.

Ingredients of Time Management

☐ Planning and organizing

☐ Prioritizing as per the importance and urgency

☐ Performing on time and as per the quality required

Time Management is a great skill, as we are trying to manage the costliest thing of our life, i.e., Time.

People who learn to manage time well, achieve much more in real life as, because of their proper planning, they do things as per priority as well as can do many things in a shorter time, thereby gaining more time to do other things.

Punctuality

Punctuality is a great quality of a person in modern era. A person is respected for being punctual. The entire Globe has become a global village now. The industries and businesses have become global now. We quite often communicate to other colleagues, customers and suppliers at various parts of the globe, keeping in view the difference of time, in various countries. We cannot be late for a Global On-Line Meetings. We must respect other's punctuality. Punctuality ensures timely action by all , which is extremely important for the smooth functioning of an organization.

Multi-Tasking and Punctuality

All of us, nowadays, are involved in various types of tasks in a day. We all have to work on our multiple roles, that we play in our life.

We have domestic responsibilities, personal engagements and professional responsibilities. We must perform our various tasks on time, to fulfil our various responsibilities in various roles.

A task, not completed on time, is not appreciated, besides, it affects our performance, reputation and reliability. Time management is, thus, very important.

Timely Investments

The value of $100 today is more than the value of $100 of future. Financial investments, planned and done today, generates compound benefit to the family. Proper investments in real estate, mutual funds or stocks, done carefully with advice of experts can be very beneficial and helpful, in future. Good Investments today can be of great help during our retired life.

The property my grandfather or even father had bought few decades back is much beyond my financial capacity today, as the cost of the land, cost of construction and property, have gone up many times .The cost has also gone up because of increasing population, increasing demand and better economic condition of the people and the country. A, 2 BHK(2 Bedroom, Hall, Kitchen) flat at Bandra West, Mumbai, which was available for Rs 4/5 lakhs (INR 400000 or INR 500000) in 1984 is now, in 2024, available for INR 4/5 Crore, i.e., INR 400/500 lakhs.

Mr Warren Buffett, one of the richest men of the world, said that he started investing in the stock market at the age of 11 and he repents for this, as he feels he should have started investing in stocks even earlier.

He also said that "Someone is sitting in the shade today because someone had planted a tree long time back." Utilising and managing time properly ,thus accrues a lot of benefit in future.

Importance of Finishing Projects on Time

Any project, especially construction related projects, if delayed and not completed on time, would cost much more in future, apart from effecting our reputation and reliability, in the market. Proper planning, preparation and strict execution are therefore extremely important to complete the projects on time. Even own innovative and discovery related projects must be done fast and on time, keeping in view own time line because there will be few more smart brains, like us , who might be working on similar projects, in different parts of the world. One should try to finish his research work quickly and obtain the Patent, to get benefit of his discovery and research.

Timely Completion of Personal Work and Work of Our Family

The admission formalities of our children's schools/ colleges must be done on time, keeping in view the admission time of the academic year. Late planning may miss the admission in the institute, we would want to admit the child, which may affect the child's academic career.

Our personal documentations like Income Tax returns, property registrations, life Insurance policies, various vaccinations for the babies, health check-ups, must be done on time, which are extremely important. Any property related legal cases also must be tackled swiftly without loss of time.

Time of this Present Moment is thus Extremely Important, we must plan for maximum utilization of time and act accordingly now, so that we do not repent tomorrow for wasting our today.

Understanding the value of time and managing the time to our advantage, are thus extremely important for all of us.

CHAPTER XVII

Value of Education. Love and Money in our life

Value of Education in Our Life

"Education is the most powerful weapon which you can use to change the world." -Nelson Mandela

Education makes a person wise, balanced, mature, unbiased, respectful, polite, and thus powerful, everyone therefore, listens to an educated man. The educated man has tremendous power of influencing people like Abram Lincoln, Mahatma Gandhi, and Nelson Mandela. All these leaders were powerful because people listened to them, followed them and their advice.

An educated man respects all religions, all cultures, and all languages. He therefore respects everyone.

An educated person is respected by all. An educated man is polite, courteous, balanced, broad minded, and accommodative. He can mix with everyone and behave as a friend, as by being educated he also becomes empathetic. He tries to understand other's problems and therefore treats everyone with sympathy, love, and respect.

An educated man is a good and noble citizen of the world. He thinks beyond his own caste, creed, culture, and even country. He is a global citizen. He wishes to help the people of the world like Florence Nightingale, Mother Teresa had done and like Mr. Warren Buffett, Bill Gates are doing.

Education changes our mindset, our approaches towards life, towards other people of the world. Education makes us positive, helpful, humble and grounded. Education helps us to shed arrogance, ego, attitude, hatred, meanness as well as transforms us into a nice, spiritual, sober and well-behaved person, who is an asset to the society.

There is a difference between an educated person and a qualified person. A qualified person may have many degrees but he has to learn to be polite, humble, balanced , matured and well-mannered to become educated.

Value of love in our life.

The life without love is like a desert which is barren, dry, endless, and lifeless or very difficult to live. The absence of love creates a vacuum in our lives. Everyone, all people, all animals need love, appreciate love and want to be loved. Love increases desire to live, it gives us a sense of belongingness.

We love our parents because they love us from the day one of our life. The love a mother gives to her child cannot be compared with any other love, or any other thing in the world.

We get love from our mother, father, our siblings like brothers, sisters, spouse, grandparents, aunts, uncles, neighbours, friends, teachers, etc.

The love of spouse is again incomparable. As like parents, a spouse also loves a lot, sacrifices a lot, to make us happy.

Love energises a person, it is a stimulant for extra energy as it makes person loved, cared for, intimate.

People who, for any reason, do not get love become ruthless, indifferent, and rude. They become impolite, uncourteous and, at times, even antisocial.

It is quite unfortunate if someone is deprived of love. These people deserve our sympathy and proper treatment so that they can return to the 'main stream'.

Even animals, like pets, are crazy to get our love. Even they love us and try to express their love in their strange way.

Love is a very big weapon or a tool or a positive way to influence others, to make people feel important and loved.

A lot of complex situations can be easily solved through love.

It is fine if people do not love us or respect us. People may try to approach a problem in a different way, but we should approach the problem with love in our mind and then, sooner or later, today or tomorrow, people would also respond with love and a nice, mutually acceptable solution can be found.

Love as a quality, can make us a happy man, helpful man, and empathetic man. It is a quality, which is not present in everyone, but an extremely good quality to inculcate.

Love attracts people, love changes opponents, and love creates win-win situations. Love can win people easily. It is therefore a very powerful quality to win the mass or our colleagues as well as work force, with whom we work every day.

Value of Money in our life

Ever since money became the media of all transactions, it became a very important ingredient of our lives. In ancient times, barter system, i.e., exchange of items for mutual benefits, was enough to satisfy the needs of the people. But as the needs of the people grew and barter system proved to be inadequate in terms of quantity and type of the items needed to be exchanged. A common media of value, i.e., money was introduced, in form of coin, minted first in China in around 640 BCE. Since then, the world adopted coins. Mohar, in India, was used in ancient times. We now use bank notes and coins as well as digital currencies.

So, for everything we need to buy in our life, we need money, i.e., currencies, National and International. And to get much needed money, people work hard to earn, as salary, profit in business or earn by using talents for which the public pays as entertainment fees.

Money therefore is extremely important, we need money to buy food, by tickets for transportation, pay fees for the schools/ college or even for medical treatments, for buying clothes, etc.

People who have more money and more surplus money are known to be rich and those who do not have enough are poor people.

The entire world is therefore chasing money, working hard to earn enough money. Everyone wants to be rich so that they can enjoy their life with all comforts. People with more money can afford to buy more costly and rare items which are known as luxury items like TV, AC, Cars etc, which poor people are not able to afford.

There is a constant race for the poor people to become rich as the rich people are known as elites of the society, enjoying luxuries of life , hence an elevated status.

But in an endeavour to earn more money few people also adopt unwanted, unethical practices, because they envy the rich people and feel jealous of them as the rich people seem to enjoy their lives much more and children of rich people can afford better food, comfort, education, international experience, etc., and have privilege to have better opportunities to become even richer than their parents.

The society is divided in three categories as far as money is concerned,

a) Rich

b) Middle class

c) Poor

Rich is again divided in:

- Super Rich
- Rich

Middle class is divided in:

Higher Middle Class

Lower Middle Class

Poor is also divided in:

Poor

Very poor, who are without proper food and shelter and any regular income.

At present the world's population is approx., 8 billion. Out of these people, about 700 million people are very poor, these people live in poor countries and developing countries located in as sub-Saharan countries, and countries located in West Asia, South East Asia, Latin America.

Few reasons why some countries are poor may be due to the following causes:

a) Geographic location – lack of water, lack of resources etc.

b) More population

c) Disturbed and prolonged bad political situation

d) Orthodox and improper economic conditions

e) Lack of modern technology

f) Unstable Govts.

g) Lack of optimum utilization of resources

h) Lack of good leadership and planning

i) Lack of proper education

j) Corruption

k) Unfortunate wars between the countries

l) Continuous internal disturbances

Be it as it may, whether a person is poor or rich, we all have to leave this word one day and we cannot take our money, assets, properties, possession with us when we leave this world. We keep everything here, our villas, luxury cars, private jets everything. Only thing that still remains with us when we leave this world is our good deeds, our reputation, people's love and respect, provided, we have done something good, we have contributed to the society, we have done something good for this world, the people of this world.

Also, it is important to note that there are also few people who adopt unethical practice to earn fast buck. There are some who cheat people and even snatch other's money. One feels sorry for such people as, in most cases, such people land up getting punishment, paying penalties for their wrong doings. The laws, eventually catch up with them and add more misery to them.

I appreciate the feelings of the Noble Laureate Dr Mohammed Yunas of Bangladesh, a famous Economist, that every person of the planet can be made rich, no one needs to adopt unfair means, to become rich overnight. His tremendous contribution as the concept of Micro Finance, was really a Game Changer for poor people of Bangladesh.

One can and should try to become rich with innovative ideas, following proper rules, laws, and timely investments. But if one does not succeed to become rich it should not matter, a person of middle class or even lower middle class is a dignified person, provided he is honest and leads a simple life.

In fact, one does even not need that much money to survive.

A proper planning about life, timely investments, preparation for the retirement in time, basic medical insurance and saving from the beginning of the career, can see us all, through this wonderful life.

Simple habits, simple food and healthy food habits, sound relationships with parents, spouse and children, few good friends, a good hobby and a little charitable service to the society, a healthy routine of physical exercise can keep us happy even with less money.

The Value of Money is limited in our life. Even richest people die and some of them may leave this world even earlier, in their 30s or 40s. They may also face divorce from their beloved partners/spouses, adding loneliness and embarrassment to their lives. Their richness may not be able to influence their spouses to remain with them or may not be able to ensure love in their life. Money, though important, has Limited use in our life and certainly not the only important factor for our Happiness and worse no one can carry his money with him when the life ends. But if the money is given to the society for the welfare of its people, like Warren Buffett and Bill Gates are doing, the effect of Happiness earned , thus by money, remains even after we are gone, giving us real value of money.

CHAPTER XVIII

What is Stress and How to Manage Stress and Mental Health in our life

What is Stress and How to Manage Stress

Stress is a feeling of emotional and physical tension. Stress is how our body reacts to a challenge or demand.

Stress can be of following types:

Physical

Mental

Psychological

Psychosocial

Psycho-spiritual

In layman's language, stress impacts us as follows:

Physical- We may have physical stress while playing football as we want to score a goal and we try to dribble past 4/5 opponent players. It is stressful, needs extra energy, and adds extra fatigue to us, in addition to possible physical injuries. It is a physical and kind of positive stress, which is self-imposed, to achieve something for the team.

Physical stress can also be caused by physical injury, due to an accident, sports like Boxing, physical fatigue from long hours of working etc, which may give physical stress.

Mental- We may have internal mental stress or external mental stress.

If we are playing cricket, being selected in the national team, we want to score a century, it gives lot of mental stress, as we want to put up a good show. It is internal mental stress.

The mental stress we face in our office, from our boss or for meeting the target on time, or due to bully or humiliation or discrimination or avoidable organizational politics, at times can give us mental stress from external source. A common man , struggling to maintain his family, suffers from lot of mental stress.

Constant pressure of parents or peers to qualify in a tough career related exam, or to do well in the career like our friends may be doing, can give tremendous mental stress.

Emotional- We can get emotional stress from someone with whom we are emotionally involved like our spouse, partner, friends etc.

The Psychosocial stress is caused by unkind social behaviour of known people like a spouse or a boss or a very close friend, etc. This kind of stress can cause lot of mental depression.

Bitter words or experience of rude behaviour of boss, friends, and spouse at times, can give a lot of mental strain. But they are also human being and can behave in a rude way, may be due to our fault. We should be mature enough to forgive and forget, to reduce stress and strain.

How to Manage Stress

Our life is very comfortable now because of the advanced technology, improved medical treatments, and modern lifestyle.

An average person enjoys good salary, good standard of living, travelling around the world, a good professional career, longer lifespan, and good domestic bliss.

But a lot people, especially young people suffer from stress. Young people are having heart attacks in the gym, football ground, a lot of young senior professionals are getting heart attacks and dying in their 40s and 50s because of psychosocial stress.

With advanced civilization, advanced technology, modern in lifestyle, people's demand of life has gone up. People's tolerance level has reduced. People do not forget and forgive easily, and quite often a small issue becomes a big issue, leading to more bitterness and misunderstanding. Strained relationships are causing lot of mental stress to people.

People are chasing success to soon, everyone wants to get or achieve everything very fast and the hot chase of achieving everything soon is also causing a lot of stress to people. The pressure of doing well in academic career and also in professional career as well as strained relationship with partners, are causing lot of mental stress to people.

Stress is a state or period of mental tension or anxiety, caused by a difficult situation which all of us have to face in our lifetime multiple times.

A child has stress before an important exam or interview, a known difficult situation, as he has to do well, the uncertainty of questions to be answered, gives stress as well as the pressure to do well or to pass.

If for any reason, we are not bothered about the result of the exam or interview, these will be not stressful and would reduce mental anxiety. A madman has no stress as he is not mentally active to think.

If, however, the difficult situation is unknown or likely to arrive abruptly, then in such situation, the stress may be more, for example, you are taking your sick father to the hospital which is a few km away and your car breaks down all of a sudden, you would have tremendous stress as you want to reach the hospital fast to save your father, the stress or mental anxiety due to unknown reason/unknown difficulty is more harmful and more serious.

Stress, at times, may be our own creation.

In most of the cases however, the stress or mental anxiety is created by us.

If we want to do very well in the exams, and we study till late night, work much harder than others; it is not stress, it is the effect of our will and determination to do well.

If I want to score a goal in the football field by dribbling past few opponents, I will have to work very hard to score goal, this is not stress but a greater determined effort to score a goal.

If I am to play a cricket match tomorrow, and I am continuously thinking how to score century, I will be stressed but if I go to field with a free mind, believing on my batting skills, I may play well by choosing the proper balls to hit and at the same time protect myself and the stumps against tricky deliveries. As I face few balls, I would get back my confidence, provided I had enough practice in the Nets, and would play well. I can, thus, avoid stress.

We can avoid stress in our day to day life by adopting basic ethical lifestyle. Following few tips are important to reduce stress or manage stress:

a) Avoid being jealous of others

b) Maintain and work towards a workable & attainable dream

c) Live within limits and manage your finance well

d) Save for the rainy day

e) Prepare yourself well, acquiring proper qualifications and proper skills to be employable and to remain relevant in your workplace

f) Avoid taking dangerous risks

g) Always remember you have only one life and your life also belongs to your parents and your family

h) Avoid wrong and unhealthy habits and bad as well as extra smart friends for your own safety and that of your family

i) Remember that real pleasure and actual happiness are only avoidable at your home.

j) Prepare yourself well and try to envisage difficulties of life or any difficult situation

k) Be bold and confident to face the challenges of life

l) Be patient, mature, and well behaved to deal with matters related to your own family members especially children

m) Try to be satisfied with what you have and keep them safe. Chasing more things may give you stress and make you lose what you have.

n) Self-contentment is the key to happiness.

o) Learn to forgive and forget. It removes stress. Let us all have less stress and learn to be happy in life.

p) We should learn to anticipate the stress and be prepared for it. Professionals have stress due to the demand of their profession. In rural areas, farmers have stress due to low yield, less power, less rain, etc. In fact, a lot of farmers commit suicide due to financial stress. We should prepare ourselves in advance, to face the challenges that might give us stress.

If we learn to anticipate the level of stress, and prepare for it then we will be affected less by the stress and may find a solution to reduce the stress by taking preventive action on time.

How to de-stress yourself

As we have seen, the stress factor is more often self-created.

If we want to do well in our exams, we work harder and get stressed. We want to do well in our profession, we work harder, and we get stressed.

If we try to earn more money quickly, we invite more & dangerous stress, if we feel jealous of other's achievements, we invite continuous stress.

So, how to de-stress ourselves?

The following few important steps that may help you to de-stress:

☐ Pick up a good hobby like singing or listening to music

☐ Do physical exercise regularly as a fit body will give you fit mind and less stress

☐ Try to help the poor, needy, and the sick people. This will reduce your own stress level.

☐ Meditate when possible

☐ Laugh as much as you can

Do things which give you no stress at all, i.e., do things that brings you joy

Try not to get angry or disturbed for petty things.

Remember, stress at young age is self-created, period of actual stress, physical, and mental, will arrive when you are old. When society and even your own people won't recognise you or would neglect you, when your own body parts won't listen to you, you would be helpless with the people around you, for whom you worked hard throughout your life and yet they may be unable to help you.

This kind of actual stress will be unbearable. But if you stay engaged in service of the poor or society, can manage your time singing or listening to music, or read some good books and can spread knowledge, love and happiness to others, you would be less stressed.

It is your life, try to be happy and laugh always since, no one was bothered for you, when you cried alone or cry alone even now. Treat your life well and enjoy. You have only one life friends, this is your time, de-stress yourself, live your life and care for yourself.

Reducing the Stress Level

The stress level rises as you become old. In young age your studies, profession, love life may give you stress but the sources of stress are quite often known to you, which means, at times, if you want to avoid, you can avoid the stress.

But when you get old, the sources of your stress may be beyond you, when you need a spectacles to read and drive your car, when the same pair of your legs, which were envy of other football players refuse to even walk properly, when your strong hands shake terribly while signing a bank cheque, when your very intelligent and high-functioning brain forgets the location of your cell phone, when you can only see and appreciate the sumptuous food in front of you and satisfy yourself with very little intake, when you are, at times, treated like an old furniture of the house which you bought with your, own sweat & blood, your money. The stress level would be very high and these kinds of stress are inevitable.

It is, therefore, very important not to increase the stress at the young age by avoiding it.

De-stressing at the old age is also extremely important as it is your own problem and you are not physically strong enough to manage the old age, physical as well as mental stress.

Fortunate people, with a loving and understanding spouse as well as good and mature children, however, will have no stress as he would be treated well and kept happy.

What is Mental Health and How to Manage Mental Health

One of the main concerns of parents at present, throughout the world, is Mental Health of their children, especially in their young age. Mental health of a person is equally important as Physical health and at times can be more dangerous, as no one apart from the person concerned will know about his/her state of mental health. Mental health is affected by mental stress and emotional stress. A lot of young children, students, and young professional executives are dying of heart attacks, committing suicides or suffering from mental depression because of poor mental health. Statistics revealed on a national TV channel in India, on 29th February 2024, that 122 medical students including MBBS and MD degree courses, have committed suicide in last five years in India. India unfortunately, is known to be World's Suicide Capital with over 2.6 lakh cases of suicide per year. Close to 60-70 million, people in India suffer from common and severe mental disorder, as per the statistics.

An estimated 26% of Americans of 18 years and beyond, i.e., 1 out of every 4 adults suffers from diagnosable mental disorder, in a given year.

World Health organization (WHO), showing concern about people's mental health, has made a comprehensive Mental

Health Action Plan 2013—2030, to improve mental health of the people of the world.

Few Causes of Bad Mental Health and Mental Depression

a) Lack of love to children due to Separated Parents or early demise of parents

b) Bad results in schools or colleges and lack of interest in studies. The child may like sports or music or something else, other than studies

c) Continuous pressure from the parents to do well in the Exams/ Career

d) Obesity and unattractive personality is an important issue at this stage of life. One crore children between age 5 to 19 are obese in India as per data shown in Times of India newspaper on 02nd March, 2024.

e) Physical and biological changes and hormonal changes in a girl child's physic come after certain age, may be 12/13 years or even early.

f) Manging menstruation or tackling improper menstruation and medical treatment, etc., along with continuous heavy studies.

g) Bad and avoidable outcome of live-in relationship of young couples.

h) Effect of bad or broken relationship

i) Bad financial condition at home

j) Teenage pregnancy, an extremely difficult situation, for a young girl to handle.

k) Effect of Cyber-crime and wrong use of Social media on young generation.

Some Suggested Remedies

1. Parent's love and care are extremely important for a child. Parents must spend maximum time with the children. At least, one of the parents, either mom or dad, must interact with the children every day and try to discern the children's stress, if any, and give him/her the confidence that he/she is most important, not his/her exam results or career. That Exam and Career, are normal things in everybody's life and due importance should be given but not at the cost of their own life. Parents, especially mom, can be of great help in a broken relationship, and especially during teenage pregnancy, which is very common among children nowadays, to look after the girl child and help the child, girl or boy, to move ahead in life avoiding mental stress. Father's strong support, love and care, can also be an immense confidence building measure to enable the child, girl or boy, to get back to the normal life.

2. Children should be encouraged to get engaged in physical activities like sports, hobbies like music etc so that they remain busy in positive activities apart from studies.

3. Growing children especially teenagers, must be kept busy with more family celebrations, should be kept in good humour by the parents and elder siblings. Children must feel that they are loved and pampered by everyone at home so that they do not try to get love outside their own home.

4. Children must know that they can confide in parents with any problems or anxieties that they may have in their life, academic or personal. They must be confident that they would have their parent's support and guidance in all problems they may have, and they will always be welcome at home, with their success or failure, because parent's love is always unconditional.

5. Since the children in large numbers are affected by the mental stress factor, all schools and colleges must organise periodic counselling for all students regarding mental stress and it's remedies.

Schools and colleges, should also conduct regular meetings with the parents to discuss about any change in a particular student's behaviour like reduced interest in studies, loneliness or unhappy attitude, and lack of interest in life, in order to take corrective measures before it is too late. Parents must know that a disgruntled, unhappy and uncared for child, easily gets attracted towards drinking alcohol, smoking, and even drugs. They may even choose wrong friends and ruin their life. The contribution of schools and colleges in a child's/ student's life is therefore extremely important. The values and the discipline taught in schools and colleges are lifelong lessons, which help all of us throughout our life. But a student must be treated with lots of love, respect, empathy and with tactful maturity or he/she may become rebellious, which may spoil things further.

6. Strict and prompt as well as matured handling of Cyber Crime Related cases, to protect the child.

CHAPTER XIX

Express your Gratitude

Express your Thanks and Gratitude to God

We must thank and express our gratitude to God for his endless blessings.

God is the supreme power who created and controls this wonderful world. He has given all of us, free oxygen, free light, free air, free water, flowers, trees, snow, sand, sea, mountains, the list is endless. We enjoy this beautiful world because of God's kindness.

He also guides us, tries to tell us to follow proper routes to success and happiness, which quite a few of us, at times, ignore. We make him unhappy by doing wrong things, fighting with each other, fighting between countries, and destroying this beautiful world, destroying his creations.

We also fail to thank God for giving us a normal life, which is in fact, is a very important as well as rare gift. There are a lot of people who are born blind, physically or mentally challenged. People who are physically healthy, should thank God for this, but on the contrary, we chase the happiness from the materialistic world. A lot of times God helps us to change our life style, our destiny. Only we take our success for granted, without realizing the invisible helping hand of God.

Prayers to God can do miracles . In real life, very few people pray to God daily. But the ones who pray to God, get his unlimited blessings in many ways, half of which, we may not even understand.

We must, therefore, teach our children to pray to God, as per our religion, culture and belief, so that they receive, God's blessings, which are extremely important for the 'Complex and Turbulent Journey' of our life.

Most of us believe in God, his creations, his blessings, his kind help, his remote guidance, and indications about what to do and what not to do. We also know that quite a few people in this world cannot enjoy the abundant treasure the God has created and given to us, quite a few cannot see this beautiful world, can't even see their parents as they may be blind, quite a few cannot walk, and quite a few cannot speak as well.

Those of us who are normal, therefore, must be grateful to God for keeping us healthy and letting us enjoy the resources of this world, the increasing comfort due to advanced technology, a loving family life, an enjoyable youth, friendship, relationships, career, and all the comforts of the world.

Most of us take things for granted as we have them. Ask a man who has lost both legs in the war or ask a man who has lost the eyes in the accident, how they miss their earlier days. They would do anything to get back their legs and eyes.

That is why we must always be grateful and thankful to the God for all his kindness and blessings without which our lives would be miserable.

We pray to God before exams, or whenever we are in trouble but if we pray to God daily to thank him, it would give us immense happiness, confidence, and strength to face the problems of our lives.

I feel, there is no time for praying, we can pray to God whenever we wish to, whenever we have some time to ourselves. We should pray to God and thank him for his kindness and blessings, the real solution to all our problems.

We should believe in God, the Almighty and try to feel him around us so that we do only right, proper, and good things in life, the secret of the Life Management.

We must express our thanks and gratitude to God every day.

One of my dear friends sent me a nice quote about thanking God, I thought of sharing with you:

'Dear God,

From the bottom of my Heart

I want to THANK YOU

For loving me,

For forgiving me,

For healing me,

And for never leaving me'

We should, therefore, thank God at every opportune moment for his abundant love, care and blessings.

Thank your parents and be grateful to them for your wonderful upbringing and their sacrifice.

Our life begins when we are born in this world. Our mothers bear us in their wombs for nine months and tolerate whole lot of hardships like ill health, lack of energy, complications of pregnancy and ultimately extreme pain of child birth. Many women have died during the child birth. The pain that no man can ever tolerate, and mothers tolerate, and goes through this pain time and again.

In earlier days, people used to have many children and the mother had to bear the pain many times. Queen Mumtaz, the

Queen of Shahjahan, the Mughal Emperor of India, died just after giving birth to the 14th child and later 'Taj Mahal' was built in her memory by Shahjahan, the Emperor of India, which is known as an example of 'Memoir of the Epitome of Love.'

A father also contributes in our life a lot. He goes out to earn the bread and butter for us, slogs throughout his life to run the family, for our education, and our well-being. The parents in poor families have a real hard time, bringing up their children. The parents sacrifice a lot to keep the children happy as they love their children the most.

So, when we grow up, we may or may not see the struggle the parents have gone through, but we must know that every parent, rich, poor, very poor, sacrifice a lot, and work hard to make their children happy, to give them good education, to give them food, and all the things needed by a child. They, at times, may remain hungry but even poor parents make sure their children do not sleep hungry.

When a child is sick, parents, especially the mother, does not sleep, she stays with the child twenty-four hours, looks after him, feeds him, gives him medicines and takes care of him.

Someone has very nicely said, 'Since the God cannot be everywhere at all times, he created Mother.'

Mother to us, is like God/Goddess. Nothing is more important to her than her child. It is the same with a father. Children are very dear to him. He also sacrifices a lot, works very hard to look after his wife and children, his parents, his own family.

There is an example in the history. Babar the Mughal Emperor of India, prayed to Allah/God, to take his life instead of his son, Prince Humayun, who was very young and seriously ill, as per the advice of a Fakir/ Saint. Babar died in 3 months and Humayun survived.

We should not neglect our parents when we grow up and become independent. We may live in any part of the world but we must help our parents, when they need us.

Children should express their Gratitude to their parents to make them feel happy. Gratitude should not only be expressed on Mother's day and Father's day, parents should feel wanted, loved, cared for and comfortable in presence of their children even when they are married.

Children's attitude and approach towards parents would enable the parents to know if the children really care for them as parents care for the children throughout the life.

Parent's blessings are extremely important for the happiness of the children, so please love your parents who are your best friends.

Express your Gratitude to your spouse/partner.

Our spouse, wife or a husband, works very hard to make us happy and even sacrifices a lot. Especially, a wife leaves her parents and own family to join the husband and his family to start a new life after marriage. She has to shift to a new house, new family, different culture, different people and stay their whole life. Even her name changes at some places.

Quite often we do not realise the sacrifices done by our wives/spouses. Male members may be working outside the house and for those wives who are not working in any office, they have to stay inside the house for twenty-four hours. They remain busy in the house-hold works and look after the babies and young children, neglecting even their own health at times.

Recently, I had a Head Surgery, and when I came back to our house, my wife looked after me 24 hours for about 3 months. She did not take enough rest, did not take care of herself at all. Looking after a patient, needs a lot of effort and sacrifice. She ensured my early recovery. No words will be enough to thank her. I will always remain grateful to her for her love ,care and sacrifice. Her smiling face acted more than any medicine.

In poor families, mothers eats after the children and the husband have eaten. At times, they remain hungry but they feed the children and husband.

Even in well to do families, the house wife remains very busy looking after the house and getting the work done by the servants etc. They do not get enough time to rest. Looking after a baby is an enormous task, and in most of the cases, the mothers remain unwell and weak because of the child birth. Yet they work at home continuously. Sometimes, they are without any helping hand and they do all the work at home including cooking, cleaning etc.

The selfless sacrifice allows the husband to work in the office with full energy and concentration. Wives, their hard work, love and care, keep the husbands happy as well as their parents happy. It is due to wife's love, care, guidance that the children get good upbringing, good health, safety and security because mother is the best teacher and the best protector. No one can be more concerned about a child than a mother. We should be grateful to our wives for their sincerity, dedication and selfless service.

It is therefore very important for all of us to thank our spouses for their love, care, and sacrifice which helps us to keep a long relationship and which makes our house, a Loving Home.

It is never too late to express our gratitude to our beloved spouses for the love, support, adjusting skills which make marriage a great success.

The mutual respect, the power of tolerance and the quality to forgive and forget are the most important ingredients of a marriage and both the partners deserve appreciation for that.

Let us thank and be grateful to our spouse/partners, and we must express our thanks and gratitude to them, before it is too late.

Express your gratitude to your Teachers, Mentors and Seniors

A teacher is an extremely knowledgeable, humble, and simple person. A teacher is a well-wisher and wants his/her students to succeed in life, to be happy in life.

His/her strictness teach the students, discipline and technique to complete the task on time, the most important aspect for success in life.

A teacher remains a simple and humble person, whereas, his/her student taught by him/her, the basic aspects, the subjects, soft skills, climbs the ladder of success very fast.

In a get together, people were seen boasting about themselves, saying I am a well-known Surgeon, I am a famous Engineer, I am a famous Scientist. There was an old gentleman standing in one corner, when he was asked who he was, he politely replied 'I am humble teacher, I produce doctors, engineers, scientist and successful people like you' and some of them rushed to touch his feet. A teacher therefore plays a very important role to build our career.

A Teacher does not expect anything from his students, even after they achieve something spectacular in life.

We all are made by our humble and simple but extremely knowledgeable teachers. The least we can do is, express our gratitude to them when we meet them. A phone call once in a blue moon, would give them lot of satisfaction. They made us what we are today. So let us at least thank them for their enormous contribution in our life, whenever possible.

We should express our thanks and gratitude to our Mentors and Seniors, for teaching us, coaching us, and guiding us during our early days, in the professional world. We should not forget their contribution in shaping our career, at the beginning of our career, when we were new, raw and inexperienced. The role of our mentors and good seniors is very important in our life as some of them were our idols, and we tried to follow their footsteps to climb the ladder of success. We should therefore express our thanks and gratitude to our mentors and seniors for their valuable guidance and strict mentoring, for our success in our professional career.

We should express our Gratitude to our Children

We should express our gratitude to our beloved children as they also love us enormously and help us a lot in times of need. The children help us quietly without expressing it, as they love us a lot.

One has to be blessed and fortunate to have good children, but we have to offer them unconditional love, as our children are the closest to us.

We must express our thanks and gratitude to our children also for their support, love and respect they show to us as they love us a lot and at times do not know how to express their love to us. The children are lovable, innocent and very dear to us. We cannot survive without our dear children. So, we should thank them for their support and love whenever we can.

We should try to ignore and forgive little mistakes or neglect, at times, by our children if it ever happens, because it may be unintentional, or may be due to own family commitments. We are sure that our children love us a lot and being matured parents, we must continue to love them, ignoring their mistakes, if any.

We must express our thanks and gratitude to our children, more often for their love and support.

CHAPTER XX

Planning for a Retired Life

How to Plan a Post Retirement Period

A time comes in everyone's life when one has to retire from service because of the upper age limit of the service. The service may be a govt. job, or a private job, but one has to retire at a certain age. This time and age limit is known to all of us at the time of enrolment in the job. Though the retirement age varies from country to country, people have to retire. The age limit may be 60, or 62, or 65 as the case may be.

Those who own their own business may work a little longer, say up to 75 years, but in own business also people would like to hand over the business to their children, son or daughter and relax after certain age which may be 70 or 75 years of age.

In present era, the lifespan of an average person is increasing. Many people live beyond 90 years and sometimes even 100 years. In Japan there is a 100-year club where all members are more than 100 years old.

The concern of old age, that is after retirement, when a person does not go to office or is not involved in day to day official duties and complex problems of the office, is that he has lot of time at his disposal. How should he pass his time in the entire day, is a big point of concern?

As we grow old, the physical activities reduce drastically. The sports, games, walk are all reduced.

Staying at home with an equally old spouse may, at times, lead to more and avoidable arguments which eventually may lead to misunderstanding and strained relationship, which must be refrained.

At an old age, both husband and wife would have more time to themselves as other work like cooking, gardening, etc., also reduce as people get tired easily. But you do not get sleep easily either. Resting for long time on the bed may create other physical problems like bed sores, disturbing thoughts, remembering old and avoidable issues, etc.

Some nice ways to remain occupied in retired life are :—

Retired Life Offers Excellent Opportunities to Enhance our Hobbies

Retired life compels us all to stay at home but provides enough time to promote our hobbies.

We all know how important it is to have a hobby in our daily life. Hobby offers the following benefits:-

1. Hobbies are a great stress reliever. It is healthy and productive, and keeps us away from the unpleasant personal issues.
2. Hobbies encourage us to take a break and we would like to take a break to pursue our hobbies. Also in retired life, we may pursue our hobbies because hobbies are entertaining, fun-filled, creative and we have lot of time available to us. Hobbies, therefore, must be welcomed in Retired Life.
3. Hobbies offer new challenges and expensive hobbies like trekking, rafting etc can be challenging, but fun, offering unique experience.
4. Hobbies allow us to explore ourselves and our talents.

5. Hobbies can be Enjoyable and Self Entertaining.
6. Hobbies can provide additional income if one masters the hobby like Singing or Playing a Musical Instruments like Guitar, or Sitar, etc. One can hold exhibitions of Sketches, Oil Paintings, etc., if he is very good at it.
7. E.g. A man was working in a bank and he liked music as a hobby. He is one of the most successful Music Directors now. He is famous, wealthy and a celebrity now, in Mumbai. There were also a few Great and Successful Writers, who started writing books after Retirement and became famous.
8. Hobbies help our transition to retirement. Many people learn music or game of bridge to pass time during retired life, remaining socially active.
9. Hobbies prevent us from wasting time and getting into bad habits. Hobbies are self-entertaining, challenging, and fun, hence keep us away from boredom, drinking, and smoking etc. Hobbies also help us grow spiritually.
10. Hobbies are like Meditation. It keeps us calm and peaceful. Helps us to connect with God Almighty. Hobbies like music purifies our soul.
11. Hobbies improve our self confidence and self-esteem.
12. Hobbies enrich our perspective.
13. Hobbies also help improve our memory. If music is our hobby, we have to memorise the lines while singing, especially in public.
14. It promotes level of energy as we try to excel in our hobbies.
15. Hobbies keep us physically healthy as hobbies make us happy, reduces stress and are entertaining.
16. It allows us to sleep better as we are calm and peaceful.

17. It strengthens relationship. Sharing the same hobby with spouse or loved ones bring us closer and helps us in lasting and good relationship.
18. Hobbies makes us meet new people with similar hobbies.
19. Hobbies makes us more patient as we silently struggle to master a new hobby, which usually takes time, e.g. learning to play Violin or Sitar, which is a very difficult musical instrument to play and master.
20. Hobbies enable us to give back to the society. Singing to physically handicapped or very old people at old age home, can give them so much happiness or teaching Music in a class of under privileged children would be a great contribution.
21. Hobbies make us more interesting and popular person.

For all these benefits one should definitely learn a hobby as Retired Life offers us additional time to pursue our hobbies enabling us to add more fun to our life.

More time for physical exercise

Retired life offers us extra time for additional physical exercise to keep ourselves physically fit.

Some of us are used to getting up early and do our physical workout in the early morning before going to office/workplace, and some of us are used to work out in the evening or late evening.

But the retirement enables us to work out in the morning and evening as travel time to office has been saved and we do not come back from the office in the evening, feeling tired and needing rest.

We can very well manage around 45 mins to 1 hour in the morning as well as in the evening for physical activities.

Additional time available for physical fitness is a huge advantage.

Quite a few of us, especially at senior position in the corporate sector/industries find less time for our physical activities because of late working hours, frequent travelling for office work, extremely busy and complex official routine. And often, our busy office routine takes away our precious personal time/leisure.

Very frequently, we see people becoming out of shape because of the extremely busy office schedule and eventually developing hypertension, diabetes, heart related problems, and digestion problem.

Middle aged people in 40s and 50s tend to develop similar symptoms because of lack of physical activities.

There are plenty of examples nowadays when we hear about smart, young, senior executives of companies dying of heart attack or developing serious physical problems at early age.

They work very hard to become successful and as they climb the ladder of success, they fall ill and can't enjoy their success, as they become physically unfit. Their family also suffer due to them. Being physically fit is, therefore, extremely necessary, and retired life offers us plenty of very valuable time. We must utilise this additional time available to us, being present at home, and as we are retired, can follow a well-planned daily physical training routine.

The time table must include long jogging/walking, stomach crunches, exercise of upper body, lower body and limbs.

Yoga of 30/40 min, 4/5 times a week, in addition to our work out can be of immense benefit.

30/40 minutes Meditation , every day, can also help us a lot.

Because of the Retirement, we are compelled to stay a home hence we should utilise every day for our much needed physical/ mental health.

Few Suggested Steps to enable the Senior Citizens to have a better, busier and more enjoyable life.

Few suggested activities which can keep us suitably engaged in retired life are :-

Music

Inculcate or learn some hobby like singing, playing some musical instrument etc. Music is self-entertaining and can keep us busy for a long time. Spending 2/3 hours or even more, in a day is possible.

Making Sketches/Oil Paintings

If you are good at drawing sketches or doing oil painting/watercolour painting on a canvas, it can be a great hobby. An oil painting can keep you beautifully engaged for weeks. It also gives a great satisfaction because of your creativity.

Gardening

Gardening is another good hobby which can keep you engaged for a long time in a day, both in the morning and in the evening. It is a great experience when you see a small sapling grow into a big and healthy plant. When you water a plant, the plant speaks to you with its happiness. When the plant gives flowers, it gives you tremendous joy. You do not want to pluck it nor do you allow anyone to pluck the flower.

When the plant gives fruits, it gives you immense happiness and you feel proud to show the fruits to others as you are directly/indirectly involved in looking after the plant and it's growth.

Cooking

We cook to feed ourselves as well as someone we love. Our mothers have been cooking to feed us through ages. Our wives have been cooking to feed us ever since she was married and came to our house. Wives have been cooking to feed the husbands for centuries. And quite a few of us always felt that it is the duty of the wives to cook and feed the husbands and the children.

It is a misnomer, everyone in the house who is a grown-up and can handle the kitchen and should learn to cook.

If we remain busy in our work, career and are unable to find enough time to cook in the house for our own family members, then after retirement, there is plenty of time to learn and cook. So, let us learn cooking and cook for our near and dear ones. It gives us immense happiness when, being new to the job, you cook something for the family and the family members including your spouse appreciate it.

Cooking is a good old expression of your love for your own people. You want to cook and feed them because you love them, the 'love' being the best ingredient of cooking.

It is therefore a good hobby to learn, if not now then after retirement.

Looking after pets

A pet, like a dog, a cat, or even a parrot can be a great way of spending time. A pet can offer us lots love, affection, and loyalty. A dog also provides lot of security to senior citizen as there are few who take advantage of senior citizen, when they are very old or staying in a house/flat all alone. A couple of dogs can not only be great company, but also a huge source of security as well as a playing and lovable company.

I remember our dogs 'Buzo' and later on 'Jackie'. When I returned home at midnight from an outdoor official trip, the dog would know that I was returning home, the moment I opened the gate of our house, which was about 70 to 80 meters away, from the building, he would start barking and he wouldn't allow me to go anywhere without meeting him, patting him and he licking me all over my hand, and face. That was his way of showing love. It was a very heart-warming experience and a great feeling.

A dog is also a great companion. He can keep you engaged very well. His presence near you itself is a very nice feeling, the way he would like to sit or sleep on your lap, or sit on your feet and move with you wherever you go. A pet's love and loyalty can teach us, human beings, a lot.

Write Books

As the post retirement period allows us lot of time for ourselves, we can utilize this time, in a very positive way, by writing few books.

We may like to write from our professional experience or anything we would like to convey to the present young generations or any social issue which needs to be written to enlighten the public for the benefit of the society.

The book can be published as hard copies or as e books.

Writing a book can keep us suitably engaged for few months, as lot of work and research work would be required to make the book worth reading.

A book is read by the people for years and generations. A good book, with good contents are beneficial for the society, would be read and remembered for a long time, even decades after we are gone. Writing a good and useful book would encourage young generations to follow our footsteps.

Help the young generation by getting attached to some Educational Institution.

A retired person is only retired from his job. He is still a well-educated person with vast experience and can serve as a 'great asset' to the society and the society can benefit a lot from such people.

A highly educated person with great experience should ideally be connected to some educational institutions. He can volunteer to take a few lectures on the following subjects, which in addition to the syllabus, can help the students in their personal and professional life.

- Leadership- A retired senior official can enlighten the students on leadership through some relevant and practical case studies of present era.
- Sharing latest industry practices of the area of his specialization- E.g. A retired Marketing Director can educate the students with important marketing tips, required in present business environment.
- A retired Finance person can educate students on Investment Management and on importance of investment which a lot of students are unaware.
- He can help the students with Internships and Placements, with his contacts in the Industries.
- A retired person , with good qualifications and experience, can be Good Mentor for the students.

If any senior retired person volunteers to educate the students without any monetary benefits, it will be a great social service in addition to remaining engaged for a good cause.

Give back to the society

One can, as a retired person, help the society in many ways. He can join any NGO and serve the people of the society. He can volunteer to do social service for 2 to 3 days of a week or whenever possible by joining hands with people who are offering such services to the needy people of the society.

Few suggested services are:

- Teaching under-privileged children of slum areas in cities and towns.
- Helping single, very old senior citizens in village or city, wherever one stays.
- Giving jobs to underprivileged young children who are school dropouts or college dropouts with own contacts.
- Helping local Govt. authorities in any welfare-oriented schemes in one's own location, like vaccination drive, or providing a helping hand during flood, or other emergencies.

Spouses should appreciate each other's contribution and treat each other with love and respect since both of them struggled through the ups and downs together, sacrificing a lot for the family's wellbeing.

Quite often retired life becomes miserable as both husband and wife fight with each other on frivolous and avoidable topics, forgetting that they still love each other dearly, they are to survive together, and they are both old. The sun may set any time and they should enjoy the available time, forgetting the bitterness, if any, of past. Spouses should appreciate each other's contribution for making the family a happy family and express their gratitude to each other before it is too late. A mature approach towards life taken by both partners can make the last part of the journey enjoyable and memorable.

CHAPTER XXI

YOU HAVE ONLY ONE LIFE, RESPECT IT, PRESERVE IT, LOVE IT & LIVE IT APPROPRIATELY

Respect your life

This part of the book is very important as we deal with the main aspect of our lives.

We all have only one life and we must learn to respect it.

We respect some thing or someone who is adorable, dear, and valuable to us.

Our life is the most important thing for us. It is the dearest as without life we are non-existent. We are breathing, we are enjoying, we are surviving because the God is very kind and we still have the life. If unfortunately, life ends, we no longer survive. Hence the life has to be respected, being the most precious possession. If we respect our lives, we will try to live up to its requirements, since we respect our life we would like to be worthy of this fantastic Gift of God. And if we respect our lives, the life, in turn would love us and we may have a longer, more comfortable and safe life.

If we respect our lives, we would follow ethics and avoid and lot of problems. If we respect our lives, we will try to be a good member of the society, a good citizen as we would like our life to be hassle free, smooth, without any trouble and happy.

Preserve the life

We have only life hence we must preserve it. God has very kindly given us a good life and normal life, good parents, and a comfortable life, to enjoy it. But if we indulge in unwanted practices, bad habits, this long life can be cut short.

If we take unnecessary risk in life like over speeding a motor bike to impress a girlfriend, and meet with an accident, the life may be cut short.

If we adopt unethical practices in our business dealings and if are caught by regulatory bodies, the tension may cause severe injury to health.

If we adopt unhealthy eating habits and do not do any physical exercise, we may develop diseases like diabetes, hypertension etc, which may shorten the length of the life.

Preserving our life, is to a great extent, in our hands. Excessive drinking, excessive smoking, erratic lifestyle, not maintaining a time schedule of eating and sleeping may cause harm to our body. If we are not conscious about our body, our life would be at risk.

Preserving our life means adopting all those measures which would help us to keep our precious life safe, harmless, happy for a longer time.

But we are all human being and 'to err is human'. We may have few bad habits like getting up late in the morning, smoking, etc. Our determination and strong willpower can still change our habits.

There are lot of people in this world who have changed their lifestyle for better. They now get up early to go to play golf, or go to work, left smoking for better health. They all have learnt to preserve their lives because they respect their lives and they want to live longer.

I know lot of people who are happy with two drinks, but there are others who want to have a bottle every night.

You feel pity for such people as we all know that after 2/3 drinks, you do not enjoy the drinks, the drinks enjoy you because you have become addicted to drinks and you may not be in your senses.

If you want to enjoy the evening with your family and friends, those who drink must understand your family get embarrassed when you are drunk and your so-called friends also hate you and worse you may cause serious harm to your liver, kidneys and intestine. You are, in fact, curtailing your lifespan by excessive drinking which is neither enjoyable nor beneficial to your body.

Let us therefore think, in a calm demeanour that we will enjoy this lovely life given by God, if we stay alive. And to stay alive, we must learn to follow discipline and learn to enjoy within limits.

Preserving our lives also includes measures taken to stay away from legal court cases, unnecessary fights, and keeping away from the bad company, who may drag us into bad habits or bad and avoidable incidents, the results of which may be ugly and embarrassing.

Preserving life means we must learn to 'sail safe', follow good people, good examples, remain alert and do not indulge in any wrong practice and avoid shortcuts.

One will be, thus, able to preserve one's life and can have a safe and happy life.

Love your life

We have only one life hence we must love our lives.

If we love anything, we take special care about it. Our life is the most precious gift of God to us. We must see that we deal with our life in a way that, life is safe, devoid of any difficult problems, kept away from all complex trouble. Our most valued life involves the following:

- Good Health – To be kept safe from any serious injury, serious accident, physical harm, serious illness, acquired from negligence, wrong food habits.

- Good Mental State – A good mental state of a person is very important for a good life. A good lifestyle, respect in the society, a good career, a happy family life, are all necessary for good mental health, which ultimately make a life, a happy one.

- A Good and Happy Family, with good relation with each member of the family i.e. Parents, Spouse, children and Grand Children.

- Good Relationships – Good relationship in our personal, and domestic life, as well as professional life are important to make our life happy.

- Our Success and Achievements – Our success and achievements are very important to make our life happy because we feel happy and proud with our success which eventually enables us to get a lot of benefit in terms of good career, elevated status, good and respectable position in the society.

- Ethical Practices – Ethical practices and honesty provide us a secure, happy and stress less shield around our life. It gives us immense peace and naturally a happy life.

- An Ideal Work-Life Balance- The present generation want more leisure time, flexible working hours in this stressful, technologically dominated, private/domestic and professional life. An ideal work life balance, giving equal importance to the family, and the work place is very important to have a happy life. There are lot of cases of divorce, suicide, mental depression, etc., It is very important, therefore, to work out a win-win situation and have a proper work-life balance.

We must value and love our life and we must keep our engagements of life to ensure that the life is kept happy , only then we would justify loving our life.

Live appropriately.

- "Live as if you were to die tomorrow, learn as if you were to live forever" – Mahatma Gandhi

- Live as if you were to die tomorrow. So many of us take this statement very seriously and go over the mountains doing everything in excess. The deeper meaning of the Mahatma Gandhi's statement was that one should enjoy his life since no one knows what is going to happen in future, but enjoy within limits.

- People die in wars, in accidents, of a sudden heart attack in the gym, in playgrounds, etc. So one should enjoy today not waiting for tomorrow.

- But in real life, God almighty is very kind to most of us and people live tomorrow as well. So if you have $1000 today and spend it in enjoyment, you would repent in future. Also if you indulge in harmful and wrong things, you may enjoy today but you may also die tomorrow quickly. So it is very important that we should enjoy today but within the limits, hoping to enjoy the next day and next day and so on.

- If we live our life appropriately we would enjoy it for a longer period of time. As is shown in the graph:

Few avoidable bad habits and dangerous sources of enjoyment that may cause serious risk to life.

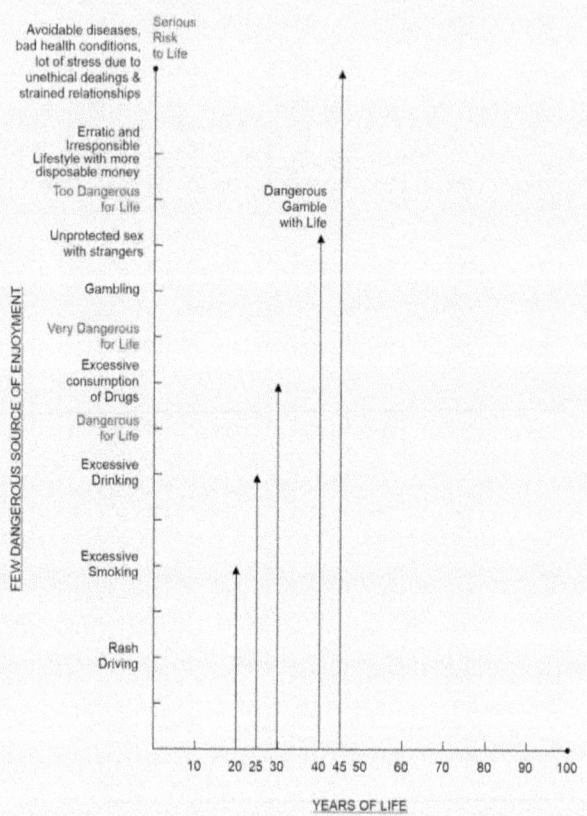

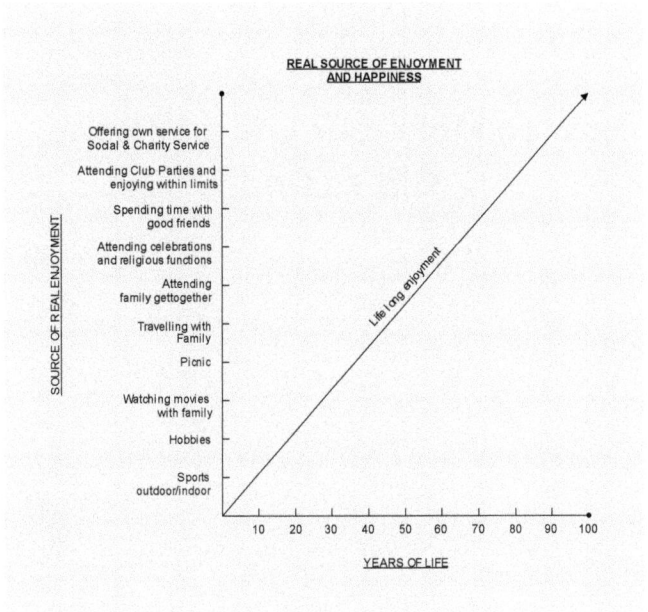

Too much of enjoyment in life in a short period of time would only shorten the life. Choice is yours.

God has gifted us a beautiful life. An average person lives till 70 to 80 years. Let us make our life, the only one life, enjoyable, glorious, happy, and enjoy for longer period.

Let us make our life useful to the society, and our country, so that we can be remembered even after we are no longer in this world.

We must therefore learn to live our life appropriately in true sense and not spoil our life by trying to enjoy it in wrong ways like being influenced by some frustrated, disgruntled and unsuccessful people.

Let us follow the good examples and good people so that we can lead a great life, and make our family, society, and the country proud of us.

CHAPTER XXII

How to Make our Life a Worthy Gift to God

"Your life is God's gift to you, what you make of yourself is your gift to God" – G W Carver

We have only one life. We can make this life worth living and a worthy gift to God if only we try our best to become a good human being and live a pure, honest, simple life with service to society and its people.

Important Aspects Which Can Make Life Worth Living

1. Values

We must follow the values taught to us by our parents and teachers to maintain an ethical, honest, simple and humble lifestyle.

2. Discipline.

"Discipline is a code of conduct for decent living in society, one with the other" F. M. Sam Manekshaw.

If we follow the alphabets of 'DISCIPLINE' and prepare ourselves accordingly, we will be immensely benefitted and can achieve a lot in our life, which would make our parents proud of us as well as God would also be happy with our hard work, dedication and performance.

D – Dream

We must dream big to achieve something spectacular in our life. As former president of India, Dr. APJ Abdul Kalam, said, "Great dreams of great dreamers are always transcended."

I – Initiative

The initiatives taken by a person are what lead him to success. We must take initiative to succeed in our life.

S – Sincerity

We must be sincere in all our dealings. A sincere person is trusted, loved, and respected for his commitment.

C – Creative

We must be creative in our approach. Creativity makes each of us unique and different.

Communication Skills- We also must master the communication skills to do well in our life.

I – Integrity

Integrity or honesty is an extremely good quality in our personal and professional life. This is a major factor for the success in our life.

Intellectual curiosity- Intellectual curiosity keeps our hunger to gain knowledge. We must continue to learn every day.

P. Punctuality.

We must be punctual everywhere to respect other's punctuality. Punctuality in global business scenario is extremely important.

Passionate -We must be passionate in whatever we are doing, passion makes us like our job that increases productivity.

Politeness – We must be polite in our dealings while communicating with others. Politeness improves our personality.

L - Long Term Planning

Long term planning, long-lasting relationships are more beneficial to us.

Law-abiding person is always a happy person.

I – Innovative

To be innovative is a great quality of a person. As Steve Jobs said, "A leader today must be innovative." An innovative person is a great asset to the society, as he is capable of helping the world with his useful innovation.

N – Natural

We should try to be our natural self. We should be humble, knowledgeable, simple, and try to be useful to the society.

E – Excellent

Excellence must be our motto in whatever we are doing.

Energetic and Enthusiastic – We must be energetic and enthusiastic to take proper decisions in the organizations.

Elegance – We must try to have an elegant personality, with our behaviour, mannerisms and nature, so that our colleagues and friends like us, find us approachable, and feel comfortable in our presence.

3. Be an Asset to the Society by adopting following qualities:

a. Honesty, Proper and Updated Qualifications, and Competence

b. Sober Habits and Good Behaviour

c. Service to poor, needy and sick people and giving back to the society. There are lot of people who need our help. Our service to the needy people makes God happy.

d. Spirituality and helping people, irrespective of their Caste, Creed, Religion, Culture and Country

4. Humility.

Famous Hindu saint Ramakrishna Paramahamsa, had said that "Spirituality leads to Humility"

Humility makes us humble and grounded. It enables us to shed our Ego. If we look around us, we will see that all great people were and are humble. Mahatma Gandhi ji was a very humble person. Some of us may also remember how incredibly humble our former President of India, Dr. APJ Abdul Kalam, was. Humility enables us to be empathetic, helpful, approachable and kind, the qualities that help us in being people's well-wisher and a friend. God appreciates such people and we all need his kind Blessings.

5. **Be a good human being:**
    a) Treat everyone with respect and dignity
    b) Do not take advantage of anyone.
    c) Be honest in your dealings.
    d) Be a trustworthy and sincere person.
    e) Be kind and helpful

Few Important Steps to Make our Life a Worthy Gift to God

- Work hard and be an expert in your field of work and be successful so that people try to emulate you and get benefitted by you.

- Perform good deeds and become a respectable and qualified person in the society and be useful to the society so that people and needy ones can be benefitted by you. Become a great asset to the society.

- Be a donor and donate for the welfare of the society just as Mr. Warren Buffett and Mr. Bill Gates are doing.

- Be creative and innovative to help the people of the society as James Watt, Write Brothers, Graham Bell, Steve Jobs etc. have done.

- Try and innovate ways to make this world more sustainable to reduce the effect of Global Warming in order to help the future generation to survive.

- Let us follow the footsteps of people like Florence Nightingale and Mother Teresa to serve the needy, sick and the helpless.

- Let us learn to sacrifice a bit of our comfort to offer some comfort and assistance to those who need it badly and make an unhappy person, happy.

- Let us adopt spirituality so that we can help every needy person of this world irrespective of his caste, colour, religion, culture and country.

We, thus hopefully, will be able to make our life a worthy Gift to God, by our good deeds, our sacrifice and assistance to the needy, sick, poor and helpless people of this wonderful world, God's great creation.

Conclusion

We all have only one life and no one knows the length of it. The life is also fraught with various uncertainties, ups and downs, problems, health issues, career related problems, relationship related problems, old age issue etc.

But we will have to go through this journey. We also know from our experience and seeing others in the society that if we plan well, take timely precautions, avoid certain habits and follow a disciplined life with ethical practices, we can go through the journey of life in a better way.

The life may still remain uncertain and may not treat us the way we would want, but if we take all measures, adopting proper habits to treat our life well, then we won't have any regrets. Even if the journey still remains turbulent, we won't be unhappy because we have, from our side, tried to manage our life well, maintained a disciplined life style, worked hard to be successful, helped the needy and poor of the society as per our means/resources and tried to respect and treat this wonderful Gift of God, i.e., our life, well, as per our capacity, with all sincerity.

The life therefore must be planned well by the parents during our childhood and by us when we grow up, to ensure a smooth and happy life.

This, one life of ours, must be a happy life. Understanding the nuances of Life Management Skills is, therefore, very important.

Many people spoil their life by leading a reckless life because of their careless attitude. They realize their mistakes later and it is too late by then to correct their lifestyle.

We have only one life, and the experienced ones know and understand it's value. We learn a lot of things quite late, and by then the life is almost over.

This book is an endeavour to make people aware, especially the elders and the parents, that if the life is planned well by the elders, the younger generations would have better, more successful, and happier life.

Everyone has only one life, but the parents can help plan the life of their children, who are innocent at their young age The children thus guided, can achieve better results in their life and can have a better life in terms of life's achievements and happiness.

This book has highlighted the importance of the 'Decider Decade', when the children are growing from 13/14 years to 23/24 years of age. If planned well, these 10 years can change the life of a child

Few skills and qualities have also been suggested for the younger generations. If followed, even a child who comes from poverty, can be very successful in life.

The book has also dealt with few important aspects of life, which can make the life more beautiful and worth living. It has also suggested that "We have only one life and it should be a happy life."

All of us, therefore, should learn Life Management Skills in the beginning of our life to have a successful, peaceful and happy life. These skills would serve as very useful guide for the parents as well as growing children for proper planning and apt management of their lives for greater success and happiness.

www.ingramcontent.com/pod-product-compliance
Ingram Content Group UK Ltd.
Pitfield, Milton Keynes, MK11 3LW, UK
UKHW020246240426
12048UKWH00027B/1636